FARM ANIMAL PRACTICE

Other titles in this series

Diagnostic Imaging of the Dog & Cat (C.R. Lamb)
Equine Practice (S. Dyson)
Exotic Species (J.E. Cooper & A.W. Sainsbury)
Small Animal Practice (R. Long)

SELF-ASSESSMENT PICTURE TESTS IN VETERINARY MEDICINE

FARM ANIMAL PRACTICE

Roger W. Blowey, BSc, BVSc, MRCVS
Wood Veterinary Group, Gloucester

David J. Taylor, MA, PhD, VetMB, MRCVS
*Senior Lecturer in Veterinary Microbiology,
University of Glasgow Veterinary School*

Agnes C. Winter, BVSc, DSHP, PhD, MRCVS
Michael J. Clarkson, DVSc, BSc, PhD, DSHP, MRCVS
*University of Liverpool Veterinary Field
Station, Farm Animal Studies Division*

Stephen A. Lister, BSc, B.Vet.Med, MRCVS
J. Clifford Stuart, BVSc, DPMP, MRCVS
*Chapelfield Veterinary Partnership,
Norwich*

WOLFE PUBLISHING LTD

Copyright © Wolfe Publishing Ltd.
Published by Wolfe Publishing Ltd, 1992.
Printed by BPCC Hazell Books, Aylesbury, England
ISBN 0 7234 1743 1

A CIP catalogue record for this book is available from the
British Library.

For full details of all Wolfe titles please write to Wolfe
Publishing Ltd, Brook House, 2–16 Torrington Place, London
WC1E 7LT, England.

Contents

Acknowledgements

Thanks are due to the farmers of Gloucestershire who have given me the opportunity, over the years, of gathering this collection of colour slides and to Catherine Girdler for secretarial assistance.

Roger W. Blowey

The Poultry section was a combined effort from Mr J. Clifford Stuart and myself. Clifford's tragic demise came in the midst of preparation of this material and most of the pictorial content is from his vast collection of slides. His attitude to the industry, his enthusiasm and knowledge helped to complete this section of the book successfully. This is a fitting tribute to the practical contribution Clifford Stuart made to this industry. His expertise and knowledge will be greatly missed.

Thanks are due to Claire Knott for assistance in proof reading and Michelle Seaton for typing and preparing the manuscript.

Stephen Lister

Most of the photographs in the sheep section were taken by us during the course of our day-to-day work, without any thoughts of publication. We therefore apologise for any shortcomings in the photography! A few were taken by Gary Hynes, whose help we acknowledge with thanks. We are grateful to Jean White for secretarial assistance.

Agnes Winter & Michael J. Clarkson

Preface

Knowledge and experience have always been valuable assets and with the constant emphasis on Continuing Education programmes, clearly the same is true today. However, the accumulation of farm livestock in units of ever-increasing size, combined with more extensive training of on-farm personnel, means that many basic conditions are now 'farmer treated'; the new graduate simply does not receive the exposure that was once the case.

We hope that this Quiz Book will go some way towards redressing the balance. By pictorial means, it is an attempt to present the reader with a range of clinical situations and, at the same time, expect an answer which provides both a clinical diagnosis and advice on the prevention and control of future cases.

We also hope that these quizzes will be both stimulating and rewarding but, perhaps even more importantly, that they will also be enjoyable.

Cattle

1 This Friesian cow (*Figure 1*) developed a swelling of its right hind leg which slowly enlarged over 1–2 months.
(a) What is the most probable cause of the swelling and its likely origin?
(b) What treatment is needed?

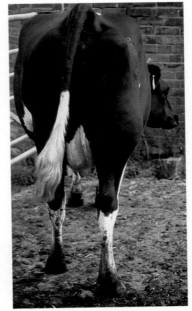

Figure 1

2 This 2-year-old Friesian steer (*Figure 2*) developed a sudden onset of intense dullness, pyrexia and anorexia, with occular oral and nasal discharges due to mucosal erosions, plus a marked keratitis.
(a) What is the likely diagnosis?
(b) What is the cause? How does it produce its effect in the animal?
(c) What is the prognosis?

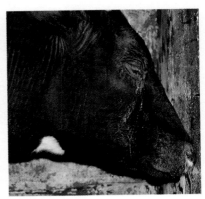

Figure 2

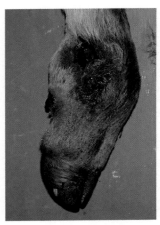

3 This 3-month-old Charolais cross-bred calf (*Figure 3*) suffered a sudden onset of acute lameness, with swelling of the carpus.
(a) What is the probable nature of the lesion? .
(b) What is the prognosis?

Figure 3

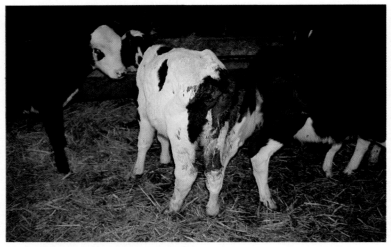

Figure 4

4 Apparently normal at weaning, this group of calves (*Figure 4*) developed a pasty diarrhoea 3–4 weeks later. Although they lost weight (the white Friesian is particularly badly affected), they were non-pyrexic and continued to eat normally.
(a) What are the possible diagnoses?
(b) What nutritional factors could be involved?

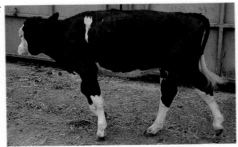

Figure 5

5 Although normal when stationary, this 5-month-old cross-bred Simmental calf (*Figure 5*) developed overextension of the right hind leg when walking.
(a) What are the two likely diagnoses?
(b) How would you differentiate between the two conditions?
(c) What treatment is available for spastic paresis?

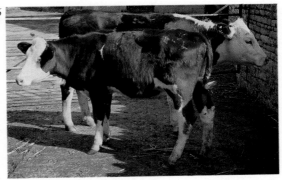

Figure 6

6 These two Hereford cross-bred heifers (*Figure 6*) were born to sibling dams on the same day and yet the one in the foreground is much smaller, having suffered periodic attacks of a mild, non-specific pyrexia, sometimes with a low-grade enteritis and depressed appetite.
(a) Assuming this is a specific infectious disease, name the most probable cause.
(b) When would infection have been acquired? Describe the epidemiology.
(c) How would you confirm the diagnosis?

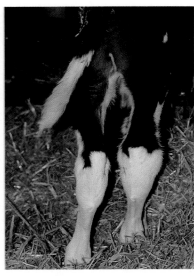

7 This 3-week-old Friesian calf (*Figure 7*) was lame in the right hind, but also showed generalised stiffness. It had a low-grade pyrexia, poor growth and poor appetite.
(a) What is the likely diagnosis?
(b) What organisms are involved and what are the main factors leading to an increased incidence of the disease?
(c) What treatments are available and what is the prognosis?

Figure 7

Figure 8

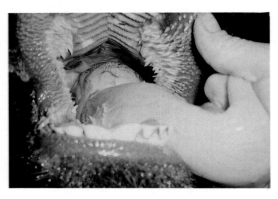

8 This 2-year-old Friesian cow (*Figure 8*) had multiple nodular swellings on the surface of the tongue, with a more generalised thickening of the dorsum.
(a) What is the probable diagnosis and its cause?
(b) At what other sites may lesions caused by this organism be seen?
(c) What treatment would you give?

9 All four teats on this Friesian cow (*Figure 9*) had developed red, raw, blistered erythematous lesions on the left side only.
(a) What is the most probable cause?
(b) Give the name and describe the appearance of another closely related syndrome.
(c) What treatment would you advise?

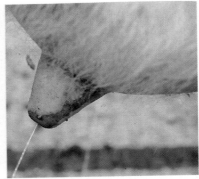

Figure 9

10 In this dairy herd (*Figure 10*) approximately 15% of the adult cows developed a transient diarrhoea with low-grade pyrexia. Milk yield was affected during the course of the illness but the majority recovered well.
(a) What is the most probable diagnosis and its cause?
(b) Give possible alternate diagnoses and indicate how they could be differentiated.
(c) What treatments can be used?

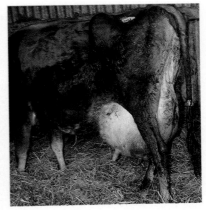

Figure 10

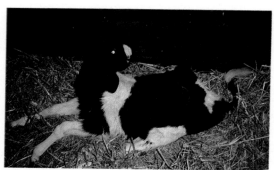

Figure 11

11 This small, 8-week-old Friesian calf (*Figure 11*) became blind, then developed ataxia, with periods of opisthotonos and extensor spasm (forelimbs) as shown. It was non-pyrexic.
(a) What is the most probable diagnosis and its main differential?
(b) What causes this disease?
(c) What is the prognosis and treatment?

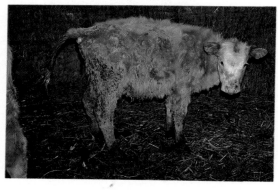

Figure 12

12 This 9-month-old cross-bred Hereford steer (*Figure 12*) was one of a group which developed intermittant cases of profuse diarrhoea, rapid weightloss and occasional mortality during late winter.
(a) What is the most probable diagnosis?
(b) How would you confirm the diagnosis?
(c) Give possible differentials.

13 This Friesian cow (*Figure 13*) slowly developed a fleshy, granulomatous lesion in the medial canthus, over a period of 3–4 months.
(a) What is the most probable cause?
(b) In what breeds is the lesion particularly commonly seen? What other sites in the eye may be involved?
(c) What treatment would you use and what complications may occur in untreated cases?

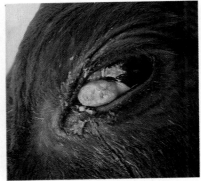

Figure 13

14 (a) Describe the clinical features seen in this 2-year-old cross-bred Charolais (*Figure 14*).
(b) What is the condition?
(c) Name one other intersex syndrome and its cause.

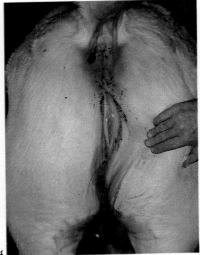

Figure 14

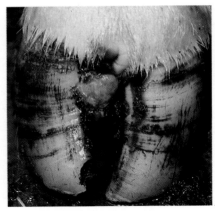

15 (a) What features are shown on this claw (*Figure 15*)?
(b) What is the most probable cause?
(c) What treatment would you apply?

Figure 15

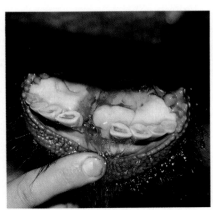

16 (a) Describe the appearance of the lower jaw in this cow (*Figure 16*).
(b) What is the likely cause?
(c) What treatment is needed?

Figure 16

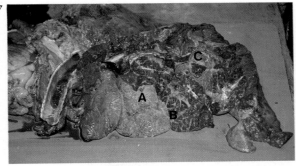

Figure 17

17 (a) Describe the post-mortem features seen in the lungs of this calf (*Figure 17*).
(b) Given that this is a viral infection, what is the most probable cause?
(c) What are the main control measures?

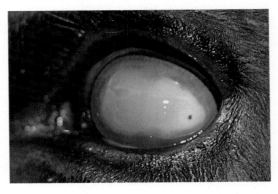

Figure 18

18 (a) What lesions are shown in the eye of this Friesian cow (*Figure 18*)?
(b) What is the likely cause?
(c) What treatment would you attempt and what is the likely outcome if this was not successful?

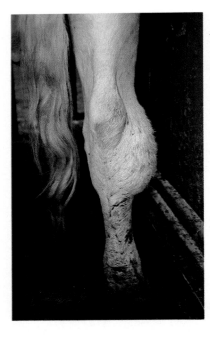

19 Note the fluctuating swelling lateral to the hock on this Friesian cow (*Figure 19*).
(a) What is the lesion?
(b) What is the probable cause?
(c) What are the likely sequelae?

Figure 19

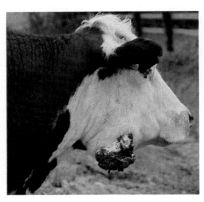

20 Note the large discharging granulomatous swelling at the angle of the jaw of this Hereford cross-bred steer (*Figure 20*).
(a) What is the most probable cause?
(b) Give two possible differentials.
(c) What are the long-term effects of the probable diagnosis?

Figure 20

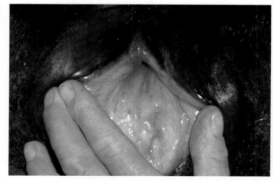

Figure 21

21 (a) Describe the lesions seen in the vulva of this Friesian cow (*Figure 21*).
(b) What is the most probable cause?
(c) What other lesions/disease syndromes are caused by this infection and what is the major method of control?

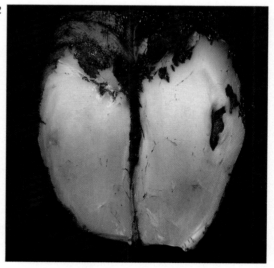

Figure 22

22 (a) What clinical features are visible on the claws of this foot (*Figure 22*)?
(b) What are the common aetiological factors leading to these lesions?
(c) What treatment is needed?

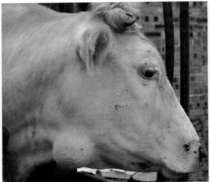

Figure 23

23 (a) What is the most probable cause of the discrete facial skin swelling in this 2-year-old Charolais cross-bred steer (*Figure 23*) and how would you confirm the diagnosis?
(b) How are such lesions caused?
(c) Describe the treatment you would give.

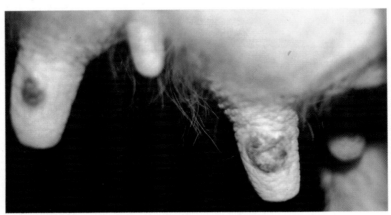

Figure 24

24 Note the circular lesion on this teat, with small, red foci in the centre and scab formation at the periphery (*Figure 24*).
(a) What is the likely cause?
(b) Can it cause disease in man?
(c) If several heifers in a herd are affected, what is the likely prognosis?

20

Figure 25

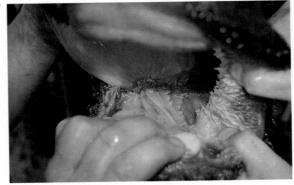

25 Note the deep, ulcerating fissure with foci of diptheresis, at the base of the tongue (*Figure 25*). This animal was pyrexic with a poor appetite, salivated profusely and had a foul mouth odour.
(a) What is the most probable diagnosis?
(b) At what other sites in the body can this organism become established and in each case how is this seen clinically?

Figure 26

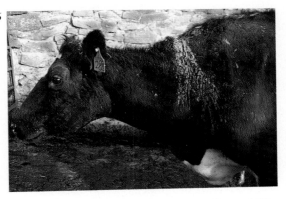

26 (a) What clinical features are shown by this Friesian cow (*Figure 26*)?
(b) What is the likely cause?
(c) What is the treatment and prognosis?

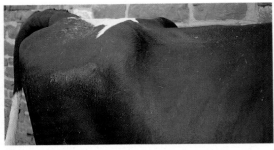

Figure 27

27 (a) Describe the clinical features of this cow (*Figure 27*).
(b) What is the clinical syndrome?
(c) What is the cause and prognosis?

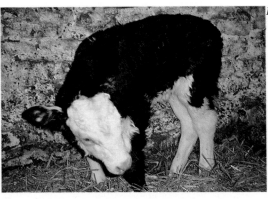

Figure 28

28 Although quite bright and continuing to feed, this calf walked around its pen with its head on one side, often pushing against the wall, as shown (*Figure 28*).
(a) What is the most probable diagnosis?
(b) What is the main differential?
(c) What is the treatment and prognosis?

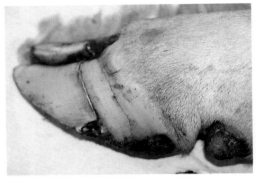

Figure 29

29 (a) What is the name of this lesion (*Figure 29*)?
(b) List some possible causes and give an estimate, with explanation, of when this particular lesion was formed.
(c) What treatment is needed?

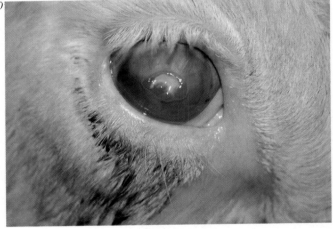

Figure 30

30 (a) What clinical features are seen in the eye of this cross-bred Hereford (*Figure 30*)?
(b) What is the most probable initial cause in cattle?
(c) List the major exacerbating factors for this disease.

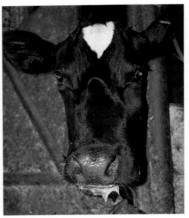

Figure 31

31 This 5-year-old Friesian cow (*Figure 31*) was profoundly ill and had a marked pyrexia, with an oedematous cutaneous swelling of the right cheek, seen especially over the masseter area and around the nostril. There was excessive salivation.
(a) What is the most probable diagnosis and the cause?
(b) Give possible differentials.
(c) What treatment would you give and what is the likely prognosis?

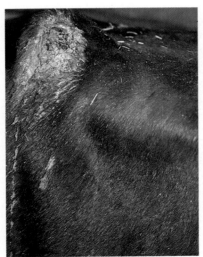

Figure 32

32 (a) Describe the lesion seen on this cow (*Figure 32*).
(b) What is the most likely cause?
(c) What other lesions can be caused by trauma at this point?

33 This cow was significantly lame, with a painful, superficial, raw and granulating area on the skin above the heels (*Figure 33*).

(a) What is this lesion?

(b) What is the cause?

(c) Describe treatment and preventative measures.

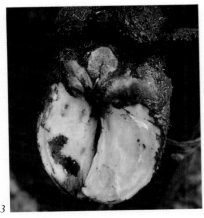

Figure 33

34 A 14-month-old Charolais cross-bred developed an acute lameness in the left hind leg, with dullness and anorexia. Despite treatment, this was the post-mortem picture 24 hours later (*Figure 34*).

(a) Describe the post-mortem features.

(b) What is the most probable diagnosis and its cause?

(c) What is the source of infection and its control?

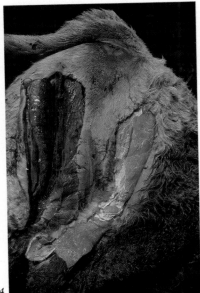

Figure 34

Figure 35

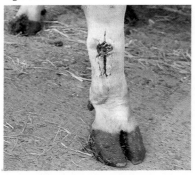

35 This cow developed an acute lameness of the right foreleg, initially with no apparent cause. After 2–3 weeks, heat and swelling were detected over the anterior metacarpal area, which later developed into a discharging sinus (*Figure 35*).
(a) What is the likely diagnosis?
(b) How would you confirm the diagnosis?
(c) What is the treatment and prognosis?

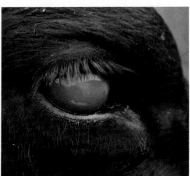

36 (a) Describe the clinical features seen in this eye (*Figure 36*).
(b) What is this condition?
(c) What is the suggested cause and with what has the syndrome been associated?

Figure 36

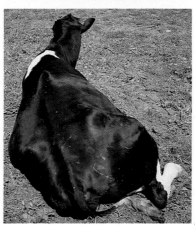

37 (a) Describe the clinical features of this cow (*Figure 37*) which support a diagnosis of periparturient hypocalcaemia (milk fever).
(b) List common epidemiological factors likely to produce a high incidence of this condition.
(c) Can 40% solutions of calcium borogluconate be given both intravenously or subcutaneously for treatment?

Figure 37

Figure 38

38 (a) Describe the clinical features seen on this foot (*Figure 38*).
(b) What is the most probable diagnosis?
(c) What treatment can be applied and what is the prognosis?

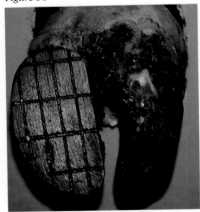

39 This Friesian cow (*Figure 39*) has developed paralysis of the left side of the face, with a drooping ear and eyelid, unilateral blindness and compulsive circling to the left.
(a) What is the probable diagnosis?
(b) List possible differentials.
(c) What other clinical syndromes have been associated with this infection and what is the source of the organism?

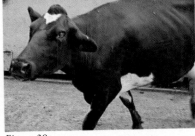

Figure 39

40 (a) Describe the lesions seen on the scrotum of this calf (*Figure 40*).
(b) What is the most probable cause?

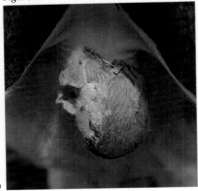

Figure 40

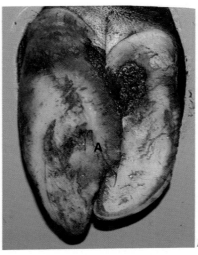

41 This hoof is clearly overgrown (*Figure 41*). List the main stages of corrective hoof trimming.

Figure 41

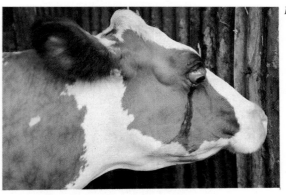

Figure 42

42 (a) Describe the clinical signs and syndrome affecting this cow (*Figure 42*).
(b) What is the likely cause?
(c) What is the treatment and prognosis?

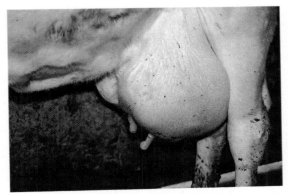

Figure 43

43 This Friesian cow suddenly developed unilateral udder enlargment (*Figure 43*) involving the left fore and left hind quarters but otherwise remained clinically normal. The underlying skin was discoloured blue and was slightly cold to the touch.
(a) What is the most probable cause and diagnosis?
(b) What is the main differential?
(c) What treatment is required and what is the prognosis?

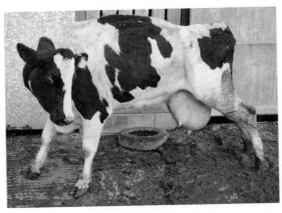

Figure 44

44 Note the stance of this sixth lactation Friesian cow (*Figure 44*).
(a) What is the most probable cause?
(b) What is the prognosis?

Figure 45

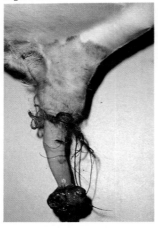

45 (a) What is the most probable cause of the large penile mass (*Figure 45*) on this 2-year-old Friesian bull?
(b) What is the cause and exacerbating factors?
(c) What treatment would you recommend and what is the prognosis?

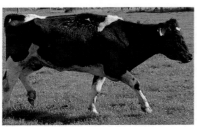

Figure 46

46 This 4-year-old Friesian cow had lost weight and moved with a pronounced stiff-legged gait (*Figure 46*).
(a) What is the most probable diagnosis?
(b) What other clinical signs could help to confirm this diagnosis?
(c) To which family of disease does this condition belong? List other related conditions.

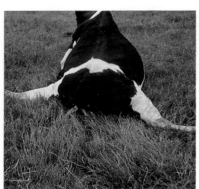

47 Note the posture of this cow (*Figure 47*).
(a) What is the most likely diagnosis?
(b) What are the possible causes?
(c) What is the prognosis?

Figure 47

48 (a) What is this condition (*Figure 48*)?
(b) What are the common precipitating factors?
(c) What is the prognosis?

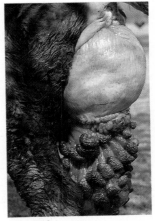

Figure 48

49 Although normally an easy milker, this cow suddenly developed periods when milk flow from one teat (*Figure 49*) abruptly ceased, only to resume as an easy milker later.
(a) What is the most probable cause?
(b) What treatment would you use?
(c) What is the prognosis?

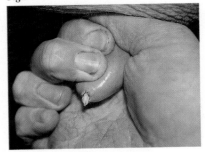

Figure 49

50 This Friesian cow was dull, depressed and anorexic, with a racing pulse but not pyrexic.
(a) What can you determine from this rear view of her silhouette (*Figure 50*)?
(b) This is a typical sign of what condition?
(c) What is the likely prognosis?

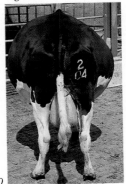

Figure 50

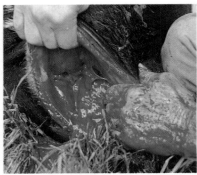

Figure 51

51 Note the profuse post-partum vaginal haemorrhage (*Figure 51*).
(a) Which blood vessel commonly ruptures during parturition and where is it located?
(b) What action would you take?
(c) What are some of the precipitating factors which lead to this condition?

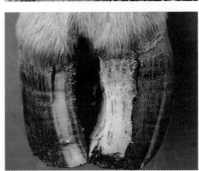

Figure 52

52 (a) Which two abnormalities can be detected on the hoof of this Friesian cow (*Figure 52*)?
(b) What environmental factors induce this condition?
(c) What treatment is required?

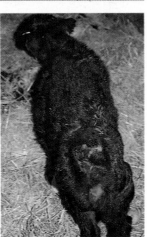

Figure 53

53 This cross-bred Limousin calf was born with a kinked tail, impaired mobility of the hind limbs and a raised red protruberance on the dorsal sacrum (*Figure 53*).
(a) Which two congenital conditions are involved?
(b) Describe the nature of the red sacral protruberance.

54 A sturdy, active Simmental cross-bred calf became acutely ill within 24 hours of birth and died soon after.
(a) What is the cause of the illness, seen here on post-mortem (*Figure 54*)?
(b) Name a related condition and state how the clinical syndrome differs.

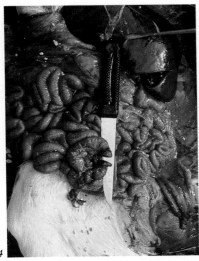

Figure 54

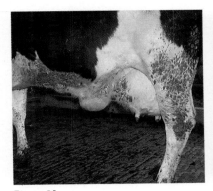

Figure 55

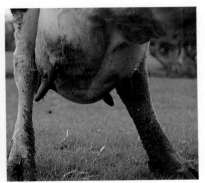

Figure 56

55 (a) What is the most common lesion producing the slowly enlarging swelling cranial to the udder in this Friesian cow (*Figure 55*)?
(b) What is the most probable cause?
(c) Give two possible adverse sequelae to lesions at this site.

56 The udder of this sixth lactation Friesian cow reaches to well below her hocks and the hind teats especially splay laterally (*Figure 56*).
(a) What is the colloquial name for the condition and what is the primary defect?
(b) Give two predisposing factors.

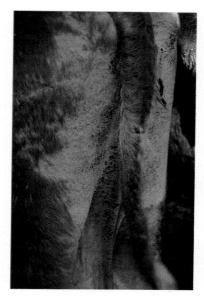

Figure 57

57 Along with several others in the herd, this Guernsey cow developed a pruritis, with thickening and inflammation of the skin from the perineum to the udder (*Figure 57*).
(a) What is the most likely cause?
(b) What treatment could be used?

58 A proportion of older cows develop a moist, purulent discharging ulcer in the skin between the front quarters of the udder (*Figure 58*).
(a) What is the name of this lesion?
(b) What causes the lesion?
(c) What treatments can be used?

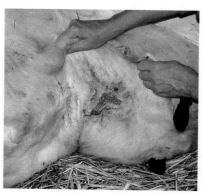

Figure 58

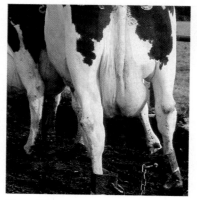

Figure 59

59 Careful examination of this Friesian cow shows oedema between the medial aspect of the right leg and the udder (*Figure 59*).
(a) What is the most likely cause?
(b) What treatment is needed?

60 The appearance of both eyes of this Hereford cross-bred heifer was identical (*Figure 60*).
(a) What is this condition?
(b) What is the cause?
(c) What is the prognosis?

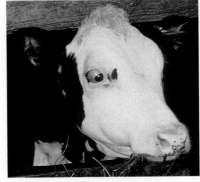

Figure 60

61 This Limousin cross-bred calf was bright, alert and fed well, but was barely able to stand without assistance (*Figure 61*).
(a) What is the condition?
(b) What is the cause?
(c) Is treatment of value?

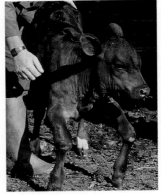

Figure 61

62 A small, non-purulent mass of granulation tissue protrudes from the navel of this 2-week-old calf (*Figure 62*).
(a) What is the nature of the lesion?
(b) What treatment, if any, is required?

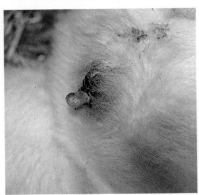

Figure 62

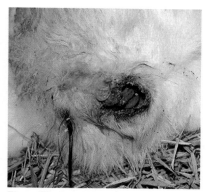

Figure 63

63 A 4-week-old male calf developed an enlarged, discharging fistula cranial to the prepuce (*Figure 63*).
(a) What are the likely causes and their differentiation?
(b) Is treatment likely to be of any value?

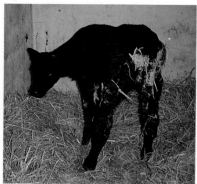

Figure 64

64 A farm is experiencing a yellow/white, pasty, mucoid scour in calves at 10–14 days old (*Figure 64*). Morbidity is high, but mortality low, with most calves being left unthrifty but eventually recovering.
(a) What are the most probable infectious causes?
(b) Give the reasons why other infectious causes of calf scour have been excluded.
(c) What are the main control measures in the prevention of viral diarrhoea?

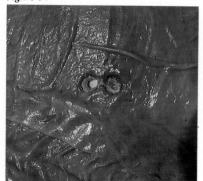

Figure 65

65 A 2-week-old calf was found moribund, eyes sunken, at subnormal temperature and in advanced shock. Note the post-mortem appearance of the affected organ (*Figure 65*).
(a) Describe the lesions.
(b) Is this a common condition?
(c) What factors are thought to trigger the development of ulcers?

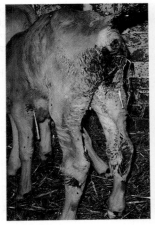

Figure 66

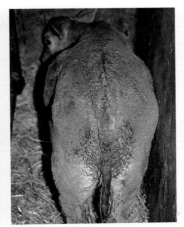

Figure 67

66 (a) Describe the clinical features shown in this 3-week-old cross-bred Charolais calf (*Figure 66*).
(b) What is the most probable diagnosis and the causative agent?
(c) What factors are important in the epidemiology of the disease and what treatment can be used?

67 This 4-week-old cross-bred Charolais calf was unthrifty, with a chronic pasty diarrhoea and often developed rumenal bloat after feeding (*Figure 67*).
(a) What is the probable lesion?
(b) What are the major causes of such a syndrome?
(c) What treatment can be used?

68 (a) Describe the lesions seen in the calf (*Figure 68*).
(b) What are the possible diagnoses?
(c) What treatment would be of value?

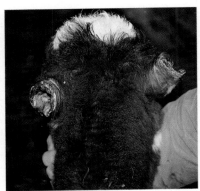

Figure 68

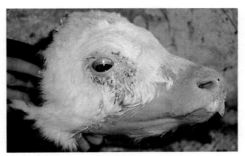

Figure 69

69 (a) Describe the lesions shown on this calf (*Figure 69*).
(b) What is the most probable cause?

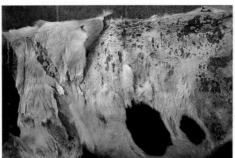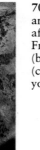

Figure 70

70 (a) Describe the lesions and name the condition affecting this 2-year-old Friesian heifer (*Figure 70*).
(b) What causes the lesions?
(c) What treatment would you give this animal?

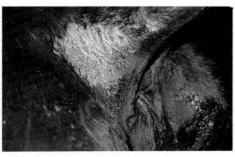

Figure 71

71 This cow has a pruritic area of thick skin encrustation, overlying a moist exudate in the fold of the skin beside the tail (*Figure 71*).
(a) What is the most likely cause?
(b) What other types of mange occur in cattle?
(c) What treatment would you use?

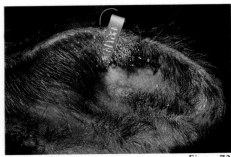

Figure 72

72 Small beige-coloured oval bodies can be seen glued to the hair shafts on the ear-tip of this calf (*Figure 72*).
(a) What are they?
(b) What species of parasite might be involved?
(c) How are infestations seen clinically?

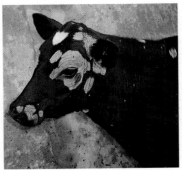

Figure 73

73 (a) What is the most probable cause of the circumscribed areas of alopecia in this calf (*Figure 73*)?
(b) What organisms might be involved and how do they affect the calf?
(c) How is the disease spread and what treatment would you use?

74 A cluster of 5 nodular skin protruberances is seen over the lumbar area of this steer and an off white spherical body has been manually expressed from a nodule over the anterior chest (*Figure 74*).
(a) What is the colloquial name for this condition and name the causative organisms.
(b) At what time of the year would you expect to see this stage?
(c) What is its economic significance?

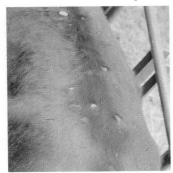

Figure 74

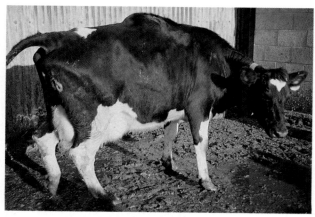

Figure 75

75 This cow suddenly developed a large, soft, pain-
less and fluctuating skin swelling over the thoracic
spine (*Figure 75*).
(a) What is the most probable nature of the lesion
and its differential diagnosis?
(b) How is the lesion likely to have been caused?
(c) What treatment is necessary?

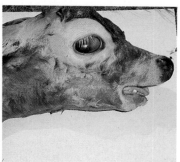

76 (a) This cross-bred Charolais calf
was stillborn with a congenital abnormality (*Figure 76*). Give the scientific
and colloquial name of the abnormality.
(b) What is the general term for this
type of congenital abnormality?
(c) What is the likely cause?

Figure 76

Pigs

77 You have been called to a sow's 10th farrowing on a 200-sow unit and find that she appears to have finished farrowing when you arrive. There are 10 live piglets and 3 dead ones (*Figure 77*). You examine the sow and can find no evidence for further piglets. The piglets have non-expanded lungs. You examine the herd records and discover that there are sows which have had up to 12 litters. What advice do you give?

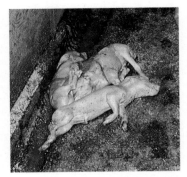

Figure 77

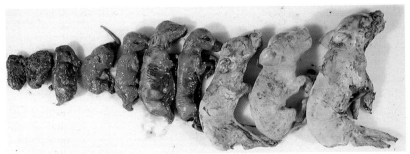

Figure 78

78 A litter of piglets contains 4 live piglets, 3 stillborn piglets and 7 mummies (*Figure 78*).
(a) What may have caused the problem?
(b) How can you confirm your suspicions?
(c) What will you do about it?

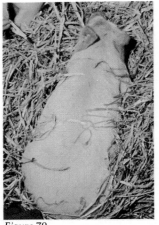

Figure 79

79 You have been called to see a group of weaners weighing 20 kg, 10 of which have developed respiratory disease. They are febrile (41.0°C) and dull. Two have died. The animal shown in *Figure 79* has congested ears and was breathing heavily. It was found to be reluctant to rise during examination and to have little tone in its muscles. Its skin developed red and blue mottling during examination.

(a) What may have caused the disease?
(b) How would you confirm your suspicions?

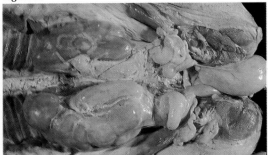

Figure 80

80 A stunted pig weighing 8 kg at 12 weeks of age is killed and examined post-mortem. *Figures 80* and *81* show what was found. Identify the problem.

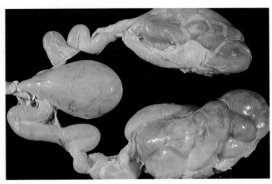

Figure 81

81 The faeces shown in *Figure 82* was photographed on the floor of a farrowing pen containing a litter 19 days of age.
(a) Why is the faeces white?
(b) Which diseases could cause this type of faecal change?

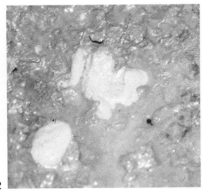

Figure 82

82 The sow (*Figure 83*) had not eaten her feed and her litter were constantly attempting to suck. They had begun to lose condition. Identify the problem and suggest what might be the cause. How would you manage this problem:
(a) In the sow?
(b) In the litter?

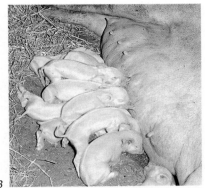

Figure 83

83 An abnormal feature (*arrowed*) was noted incidentally in the carcase in *Figure 84*. Identify it and describe the significance of this abnormality in:
(a) A pig intended for slaughter.
(b) One intended for breeding.

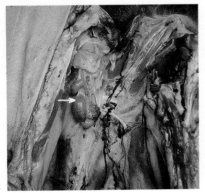

Figure 84

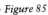
Figure 85

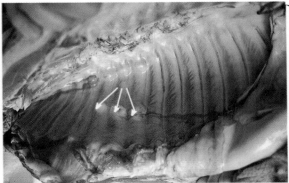

84 Identify the feature found incidentally at slaughter in the pig in *Figure 85* (*arrows*). What action might you consider if several animals were affected?

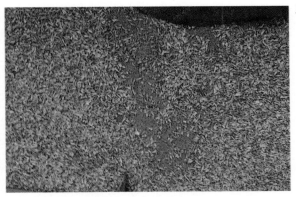
Figure 86

85 Pigs were found to refuse food after food was taken from a bin which had been disused for a month. *Figure 86* illustrates the appearance of the meal concerned. What is the reason for the food refusal?

Figure 87

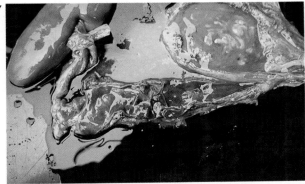

86 The organs shown in *Figure 87* were taken from a gilt which died 7 days after service. She was seen to be ill the previous evening and was treated with intramuscular penicillin. She was housed in a slatted sow stall in well-lit conditions and no reason for her illness was identified at the time. It was ascribed, by the owner, to pneumonia which had occurred in the group of gilts concerned.

(a) Identify the cause of the problem and say how you would confirm its presence.

(b) What could you do to prevent further cases in other gilts?

Figure 88

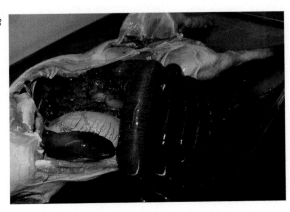

87 Examination of a 30 kg pig which had died suddenly revealed the features seen in *Figure 88*. Identify the cause of death.

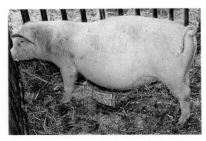

88 Identify the condition affecting the 14-week-old whey-fed pig shown in *Figure 89*. Suggest a possible cause for the condition. The terminal ileum of the same pig is shown in *Figure 90*.

Figure 89

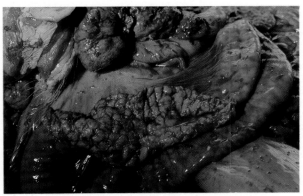

Figure 90

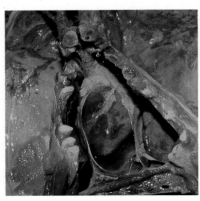

89 Note the appearance of the heart of a piglet (*Figure 91*). It died suddenly at 10 days of age. No other animal in the litter was affected. What might be the cause?

Figure 91

90 This 4-day-old piglet (*Figure 92*) was found dead in the farrowing pen. The cause of death recorded by the pigman was 'overlain'. Do you think this is correct?

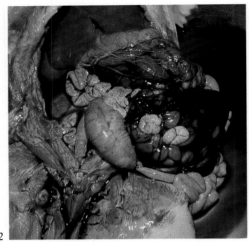

Figure 92

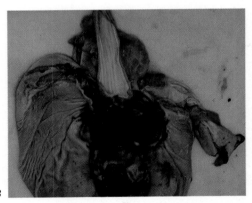

Figure 93

91 The pig from which this stomach was taken weighed 50 kg and had died suddenly. The carcase was pale and the stomach contents appeared to consist largely of rubbery black material. When the mucosa was washed it appeared as illustrated in *Figure 93*.
(a) What was the cause of death?
(b) Would the pig have survived, if treated?

Figure 94

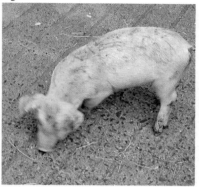

92 The pig (*Figure 94*) was from a group weighing 20 kg. All were covered in faeces and were obviously hairy. None had a fever. A representative member of the group was killed and the changes seen in the colon are shown in *Figure 95*. No other changes were seen in the carcase.
(a) What is the cause of the problem?
(b) How would you treat it?

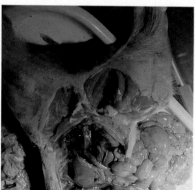

Figure 95

93 *Figure 96* shows the carcase of a 3-week-old piglet which died 3 days after castration.
(a) What is the cause of death?
(b) What would you do about it?

Figure 96

94 You are showing a pigman how to distinguish between a pig which has died *in utero* and one which has breathed. Both the animals shown here (*Figures* 97 and 98) have gelatinous 'slippers' on the feet, fleshy umbilical cords and were apparently covered with membrane. The lungs behave differently in water (*Figure* 99). Which piglet died before birth and never breathed – was it the piglet in:
(a) *Figure* 97?
(b) *Figure* 98?

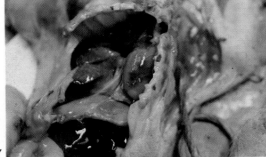

Figure 97

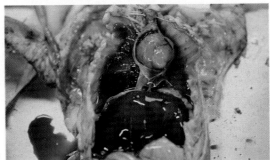

Figure 98

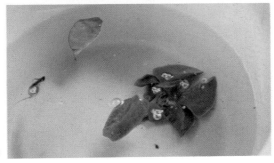

Figure 99

95 A farmer asks you to visit a herd of pigs in which some growing animals have died from paralysis. You examine the dead pigs and find that they are thin and that there is a dip in the back just behind the shoulder. You examine the remainder of the group (*Figure 100*) and find that many of them are also affected. Examination of the sawn carcases indicates that the spinal curvature has led to narrowing of the vertebral canal (*Figure 101*) and in one case to rupture of blood vessels in the spinal cord. What may be the cause?

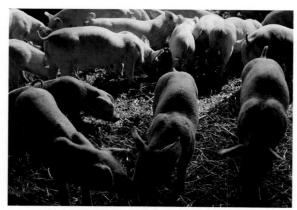

Figure 100

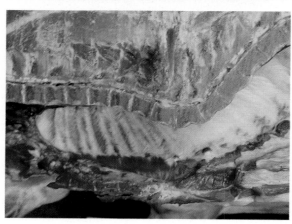

Figure 101

96 Weaned pigs weighing 30 kg were not thriving. When examined some were seen to be redder than others and some were seen to scratch (*Figure 102*). When the herd was examined some sows were found to have excess wax in the ears and some store pigs to have skin lesions such as those shown in *Figure 103*.
(a) What is your diagnosis?
(b) How would you confirm it?

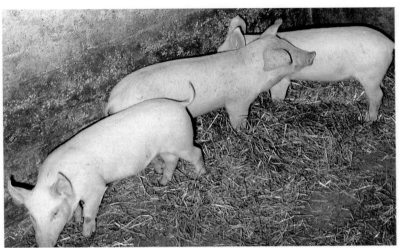

Figure 102

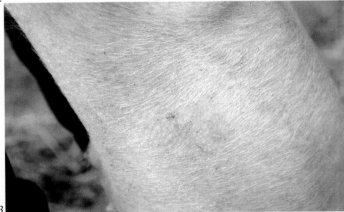

Figure 103

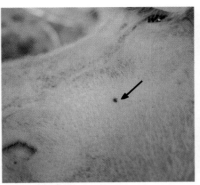

Figure 104

97 You are examining a sow which is inappetant and notice something moving on its face (*arrowed*) (*Figure 104*). The animal seems restless and has been scratching, as there are excoriations on its flank.
(a) What do you think this incidental problem might be?
(b) How would you confirm your suspicions and treat it?

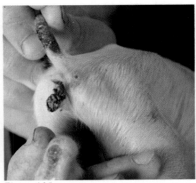

Figure 105

98 Identify the problem which is affecting the female piglet shown in *Figure 105*.
(a) What may be the cause of the change?
(b) What may be the consequences?

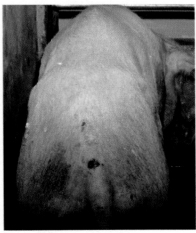

Figure 106

99 A 200 sow unit is producing only 19 pigs per sow per year in spite of weaning at 3 weeks. You examine the records and find that the mean litter size is low (10.0 born alive). After examining the records further you note that the second litter is smaller than the first and averages 9.0 piglets born alive. You suspect poor sow conditions and ask to see the sows. *Figure 106* shows a typical recently-weaned gilt.
(a) What is the problem?
(b) How would you correct it?

100 The 25 kg pigs shown in *Figure 107* were placed in a pen previously used for animals bought from a market and finished 3 months earlier. The pen was not cleaned, but fresh straw was added. The animals were breathing rapidly but were afebrile. One was killed and the lungs are shown in *Figure 108* and the liver in *109*. What was wrong with the animals?

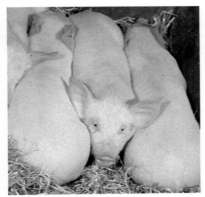

Figure 107

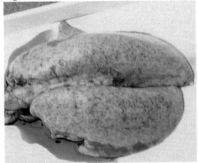

Figure 108

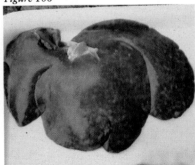

Figure 109

Figure 110

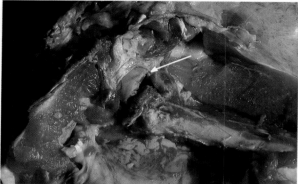

101 A finishing pig has gone off its legs. The animal is afebrile and you suspect a fracture. The animal is slaughtered on farm and you investigate the affected leg. The hip joint is exposed and the findings are presented in *Figure 110* (*arrowed*). What was the cause of the lameness?

Figure 111

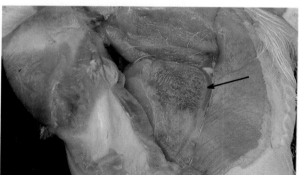

102 A heavily-muscled finishing pig weighing 85 kg has died on a hot day. The post-mortem was carried out almost immediately and few changes were seen. The skin was mottled with red and blue discoloration, there was some excess fluid in the pericardium and the lungs were oedematous. Examination of the muscles revealed several areas of the type shown in *Figure 111* (*arrowed*), a cross section of the ham. What was the probable cause of death?

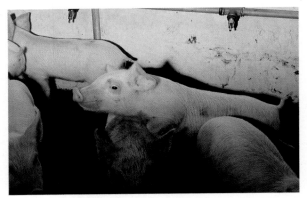

Figure 112

103 Weaned pigs are dying 10–15 days after weaning in a flat deck in a gas-heated prefabricated unit. Typical animals are seen in *Figure 112*. The animals appear dirty and the skins are warm to the touch and sticky with a mixture of sebum and serum. Not all pigs are affected, and none appear sufficiently severely affected to sacrifice for examination. Examination of the sucking animals reveals some with the appearance shown in *Figure 113*. At postmortem examination oedema of the skin and adjacent lymph nodes was seen and pale streaks were seen in the kidney medulla.
(a) What is the condition?
(b) How would you treat and prevent it?

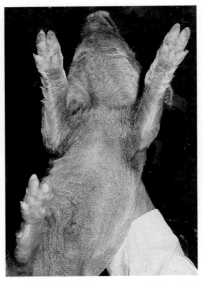

Figure 113

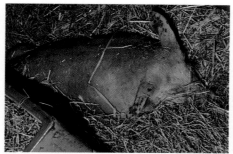

Figure 114

104 A finishing pig in a large piggery feeding swill and buying in its pigs from a number of sources has recently lost weight and become jaundiced (*Figure 114*). When examined it is found to have congestion, jaundice and to be depressed but afebrile. It is killed and the carcase is found to be jaundiced. There are no abnormalities of the thoracic or abdominal cavities, so the liver is removed (*Figure 115*) and the intestine is opened and adult ascarid worms found. What was the cause of the jaundice?

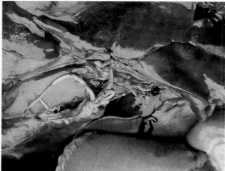

Figure 115

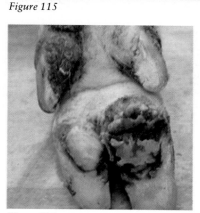

Figure 116

105 A sow kept on soft bedding is seen to be lame. She is able to walk and is sent for slaughter. The foot is found to have the lesion shown in *Figure 116*.
(a) What was the cause of the lameness?
(b) How might it be prevented?

106 The pig shown in *Figure 117* was one of a group of 9-week-old animals kept in a verandah house. All were thin, hairy and pale. One died and the ileum was thickened and pale and the mucosa was ridged (*Figure 118*).
(a) Identify the disease.
(b) How would you treat it?

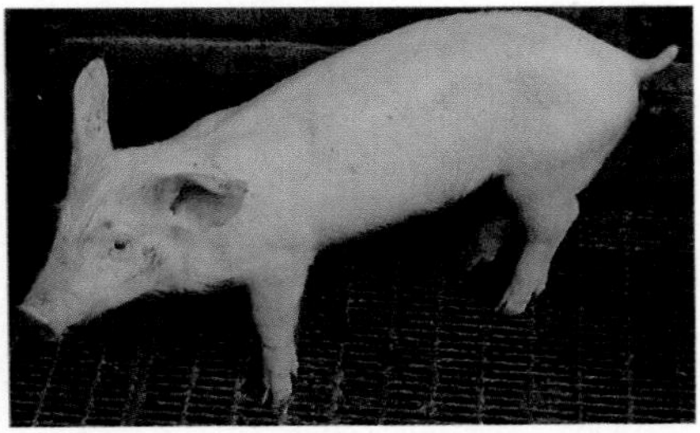

Figure 117

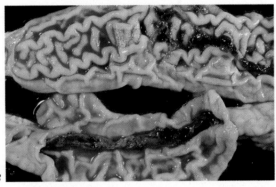

Figure 118

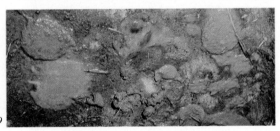

Figure 119

107 A group of pigs in a verandah house on an 800 sow unit has developed a diarrhoea which is being treated with chlortetracycline in the drinking water. You approach the unit past the dunging areas and see diarrhoea which appears to be mucoid and yellow in colour. You cannot decide exactly what the problem is, so you go inside to examine the pigs. The faeces you see inside is shown in *Figure 119*. What is the disease?

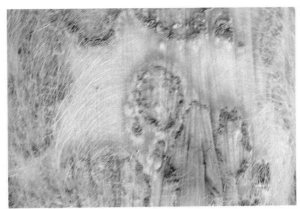

Figure 120

108 A group of 30 kg pigs is being examined upon arrival at a feeding farm. One is found to have markings on its abdomen. They are shown close-up in *Figure 120*.
(a) What is the cause?
(b) What is its significance?

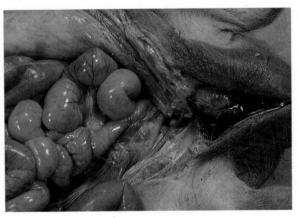

Figure 121

109 A weaned pig of 22 kg dies unexpectedly and is found to have a blackened area in the inguinal region. The swollen area is incised and is shown in *Figure 121*. What was the cause of death?

110 The sow shown in *Figure 122* is part of a group multiple suckling their litters to 6 weeks of age. Comment on her condition.

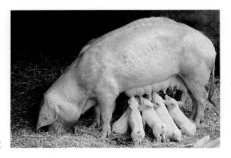

Figure 122

111 *Figure 123* shows the uterus of a pig which was seen in difficulty farrowing 12 hours previously, and from which 4 dead piglets were removed manually. No more could be felt. She died and this uterus was removed within half an hour of death. What is your diagnosis?

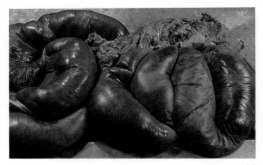

Figure 123

112 The colon shown in *Figure 124* was removed from a 40 kg pig which had died from chronic diarrhoea after an outbreak of 'colitis'. There were no abnormalities in the thoracic organs or in the small intestine, but the large intestinal contents were fluid and the mucosa was roughened and lumpy. What is your diagnosis?

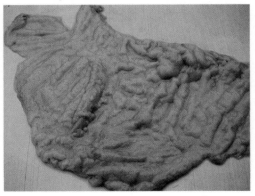

Figure 124

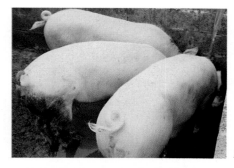

113 These 3 gilts (*Figure 125*) are housed in a traditional pig sty with an iron ring feeder/drinker as their only source of water. They are given water. What does their behaviour indicate?

Figure 125

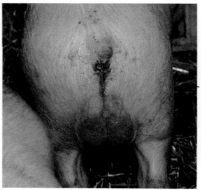

114 The pigs in *Figures 126* and *127* were part of a group of 70 kg finishers with chronic swine dysentery housed in deep straw in conditions of poor hygiene. The pigs were treated with tiamulin in feed at high concentration. Three days after the beginning of treatment, several had the reddening of the scrotum and perineum shown.
(a) What is the condition?
(b) What should be done?

Figure 126

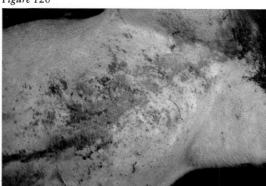

Figure 127

115 The piece of gut shown in *Figure 128* was found in a pouch on the ventral surface of the abdomen of a 60 kg pig which had died 'suddenly'. What do you think was the cause?

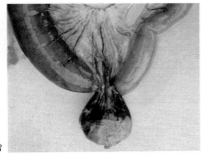

Figure 128

116 Why should the piglet in *Figure 129* be bleeding?

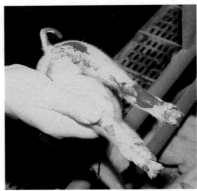

Figure 129

117 The group of outdoor sows shown in *Figure 130* have been provided with a facility essential for their welfare in hot weather. What is it?

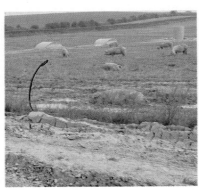

Figure 130

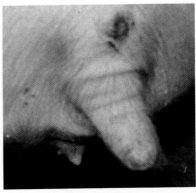

118 The stalled sow shown in *Figure 131* has a lesion on the tailhead.
(a) What do you think could have caused it?
(b) What would you advise?

Figure 131

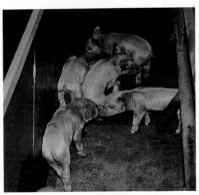

119 You are visiting a farrowing house and see a litter of very depressed pigs covered with green dye (*Figure 132*). What do you do?

Figure 132

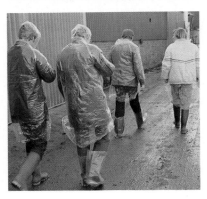

120 The people shown in *Figure 133* are wearing plastic overcoats, boots or overshoes belonging to the farm. Why?

Figure 133

Figure 134

121 The pig shown in *Figure 134* is from a group which have suddenly developed severe lameness. Some will not rise, others walk only with difficulty, grunting as they do so and one or two squeal loudly when made to walk. When the feet are examined, the coronary bands of the hooves are found to be blanched and swollen.
(a) What is the disease?
(b) What do you do?

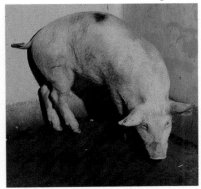

122 An outbreak of swine dysentery has occurred on this feeding unit (*Figure 135*). Pigs in one pen on each side of this scraper-cleaned house have been affected. How do you treat and control the disease?

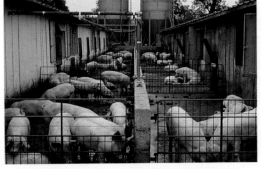

Figure 135

123 The pig shown in *Figure 136* weighed 85 kg and died suddenly. The thorax has been opened. Suggest a cause of death.

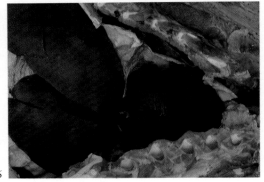

Figure 136

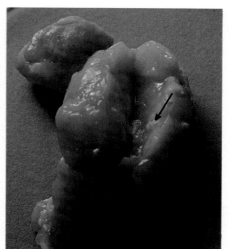

Figure 137

124 The cervical lymph node shown in *Figure 137* was taken from a pig at meat inspection. It contained small (2–4 mm) whitish gritty granular nodules (*arrowed*). What might be the cause?

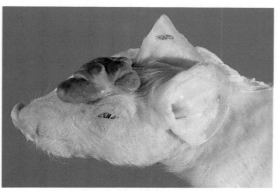

Figure 138

125 Name the condition shown in *Figure 138*. The animal is new born.

Figure 139

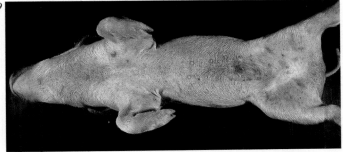

126 A 3-week-old piglet has died. It was one of the largest in a litter of an old sow on a small farm. There are two other animals affected. Both have normal rectal temperatures. *Figures 139–142* show features found at post-mortem.
(a) What is the disease?
(b) What would you do?

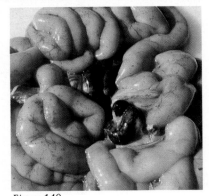

Figure 140

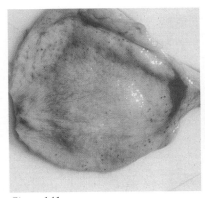

Figure 141

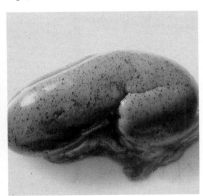

Figure 142

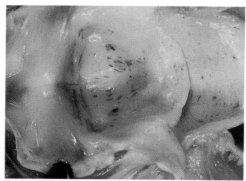

Figure 143

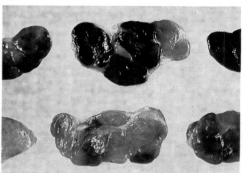

Figure 144

127 An outdoor unit occupying a field with a busy picnic spot on one boundary reports that some animals have died. Upon inspection, 5 dead sows are found with various degrees of congestion of the extremities. Survivors from the affected group have difficulty in walking and some show crossing of the legs when disturbed. Affected animals are found to have a high fever (41.5°C) and some of them are reluctant to rise and have congestion of the extremities, skin haemorrhages and conjunctival discharge. There is a convenient concrete pad at one side of the enclosure out of sight of the road. A post-mortem examination of one of the dead sows is carried out. The carcase is haemorrhagic and the spleen is enlarged. The epiglottis (*Figure 143*), the mesenteric lymph nodes (*Figure 144*) and the bladder mucosa (*Figure 145*) are shown.

(a) What is the diagnosis?

(b) What is the correct course of action?

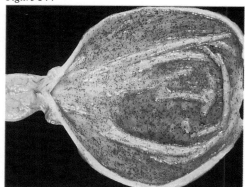

Figure 145

128 A sow has severe congestion of the extremities and is reluctant to rise. She has a subnormal temperature and examination of the chest reveals murmurs. She is slaughtered and her heart is shown in *Figure 146*.
(a) What is your diagnosis?
(b) What could cause the problem?

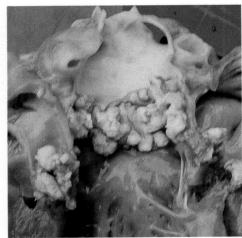

Figure 146

129 These large expanding brownish areas were seen on the skin of a weaned pig (*Figure 147*). They were non-irritant and the surface could be scraped clean with difficulty. What is your diagnosis?

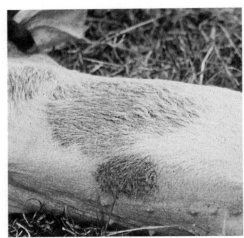

Figure 147

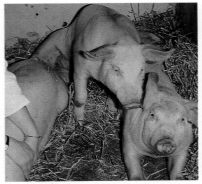

Figure 148

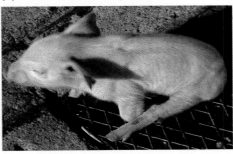

Figure 149

130 The finishing pigs shown in *Figure 148* were found dazed, one was paralysed and another had died. There was no obvious reason for the problem. The animals were afebrile, and the paralysed animal had sensation and lower motor neurone reflexes in its limbs. A broken back was diagnosed. The dead animal was examined and there was pulmonary oedema and little else. Examination of the bones showed the presence of fractures in the scapula (*Figure 149*) and there was vertebral collapse.
(a) What is your diagnosis?
(b) What action would you take?

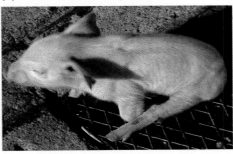

Figure 150

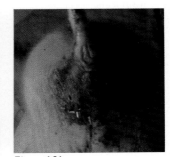

Figure 151

131 The piglet shown in *Figures 150* and *151* is 4 days old and cannot walk. It has been dragging itself around on its perineum and has excoriated the root of the tail. When placed on the ground it adopts the position shown in *Figure 150*.
(a) What is your diagnosis?
(b) What advice would you give to overcome the problems?

Figure 152

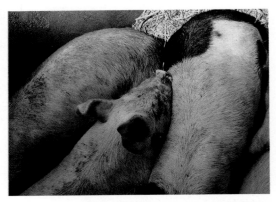

132 A group of pigs from an outdoor herd is weaned, reared for 4 weeks and then sold. The purchaser notices that some are stunted and have short noses. A few of the animals are shown in *Figure 152*. When the apposition of the teeth is examined (*Figure 153*), shortening of the upper jaw is seen. At post-mortem examination a snout section is taken with the results shown in *Figure 154*.

(a) What is the problem?

(b) What advice will you give the purchaser?

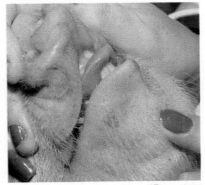

Figure 153

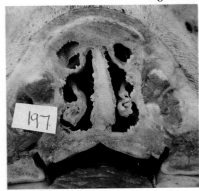

Figure 154

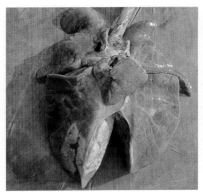

Figure 155

133 The lungs shown in *Figure 155* are from a 10-week-old pig which has died in a weaner pool. Other animals have high rectal temperatures (40.5–41.5°C) and have raised respiratory rates.
(a) Which disease has it died from?
(b) How would you treat and prevent the condition?

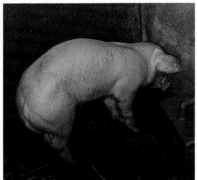

Figure 156

134 The pig shown in *Figure 156* was affected by pleuropneumonia and failed to eat or drink for 2 days. Parenteral treatment was given and it recovered sufficiently to seek feed and water. The effects of pleuropneumonia gradually disappeared, but the animal was blind and, if disturbed, would fall and have convulsions. It was afebrile when this picture was taken and was gradually recovering but still had to be made to drink.
(a) What is your diagnosis?
(b) How could you confirm it?

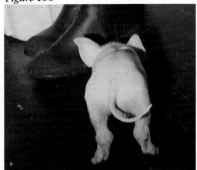

Figure 157

135 The piglet shown in *Figure 157* is 10 days old and has been lame with swelling of the hock joints for 3 days. It has a rectal temperature of 40°C. Two other piglets are affected in the same litter.
(a) What is the disease?
(b) What is the most likely cause?

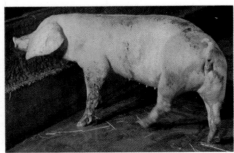

Figure 158

136 The pig shown in *Figure 158* is from a unit fed on bakery waste. Some pigs were ataxic, some were walking with a goos-stepping action and some were apparently normal, although all had dirty skins.
(a) What is the problem?
(b) What can you do about it?

137 On a visit to a small herd a few pigs are seen to be hairy and to have dark skin lesions 1–2 cm in diameter on the belly and thighs (*Figure 159*).
(a) What is the condition?
(b) What can you do about it?

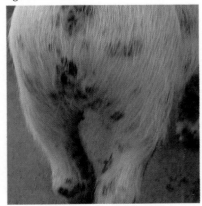

Figure 159

138 The piglet shown in *Figure 160* died at 2 weeks of age from lesions resulting from a husbandry practice carried out at birth.
(a) What is the condition?
(b) Why does it develop?

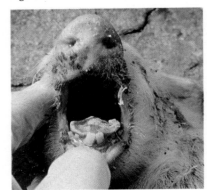

Figure 160

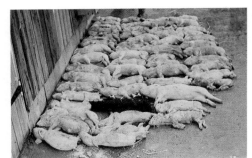

Figure 161

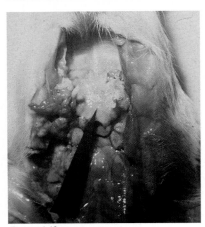

Figure 162

139 An outbreak of sneezing in sows, abortions, mummified foetuses and deaths in piglets occurs on a 270 sow unit. Other animals such as the farm cat (*Figure 161*) and the farm dog are affected. Affected piglets show nervous signs including convulsions. When dead pigs are examined post-mortem, necrosis of the tonsils is seen (*Figure 162*) and necrotic foci are present in the intestine (*Figure 163*) and liver.
(a) Identify the disease.
(b) What would you do about it?

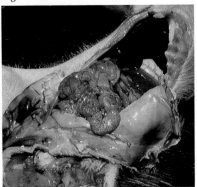

Figure 163

140 The 4-day-old piglet shown in *Figure 164* is one of 8 trembling piglets in a litter which also contained 2 normal animals and 3 stillborn animals. One affected animal is killed and the only gross abnormality found is cerebellar hypoplasia.
(a) What do you suspect?
(b) What should you do about it?

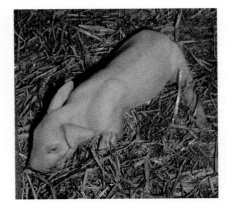

Figure 164

Figure 165

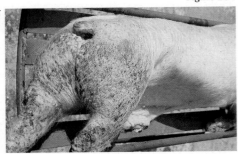

141 The 70 kg finisher shown in *Figure 165* was part of a group fed on dry meal from salt-glazed earthenware troughs. They developed diarrhoea and symmetrical non-irritant lesions developed on the skin of this animal. The lesions are dry and have very little exudate (*Figure 166*).
(a) Identify the condition.
(b) Outline a method of treatment.

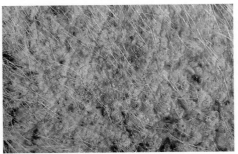

Figure 166

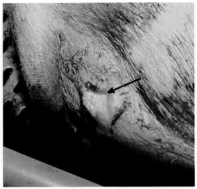

142 A 400 sow herd has a problem with vaginal discharge. The discharge begins as a normal blood-stained lochia and then persists as a purulent whitish discharge (*arrowed*) (*Figure 167*) for up to 10 days. The weaning to service interval is 8 days and it is suspected that the discharge is connected. How might you test this hypothesis?

Figure 167

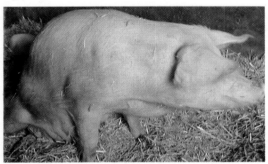

Figure 168

143 The gilt shown in *Figure 168* has been lactating for nearly 6 weeks in a traditional system. She has become unable to rise. She has sensation in the hindlimbs and a motor response suggesting that there is no pathological fracture of the spine. What may be the problem?

144 Name the breed to which this UK pig (*Figure 169*) belongs and suggest some problems which might arise in an animal kept outdoors in a relatively small pen with other pigs.

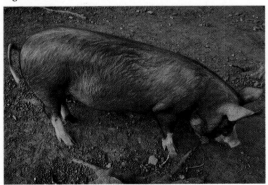

Figure 169

145 The lesions shown in *Figure 170* were found in the lungs of a slaughtered pig from a high health herd. Identify them and suggest ways of eradicating the infection from the herd.

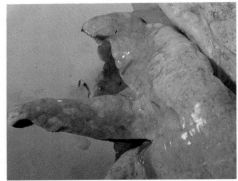
Figure 170

146 A 160 sow herd with breeding stock from all major UK companies is suffering from sudden deaths in the older pigs in the flat deck. Few if any clinical signs have been noted and all animals appear normal when inspected. A carcase is examined and the only abnormalities noted are slight congestion of the lymph nodes and one or two strands of fibrin between the lungs and the thoracic wall (*Figure 171*). The brain is found to have the histological appearance seen in *Figure 172* and a profuse culture of a weakly haemolytic coccus is isolated.

(a) What is the disease?
(b) What would you advise the farmer to do?

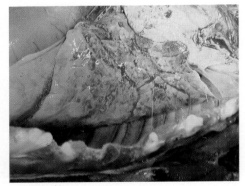
Figure 171

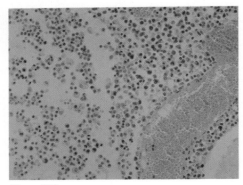
Figure 172

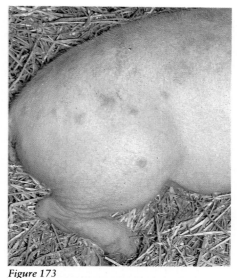

Figure 173

147 A finishing pig is lame, is reluctant to stand and is off its feed. It has a rectal temperature of 41.5°C and the skin lesions shown in *Figure 173*. Upon post-mortem examination the hip joints are found to contain clear fluid and the spleen and kidneys are enlarged compared with unaffected controls (the affected spleen and kidney are top in *Figure 174*),
(a) What do you think is the problem?
(b) How would you treat and prevent it?

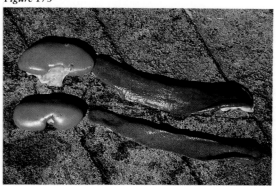

Figure 174

148 An animal in a flat deck is biting the tail of another animal.
(a) Which factors may cause a pig to begin tail biting?
(b) How may it be prevented?

149 Ryegrass pasture is being topped by a mower on an outdoor pig unit in late July. Why?

150 An outbreak of paroxysmal sneezing has developed amongst piglets 7–14 days of age in the farrowing rooms of a high health herd. The owner is concerned that it might be atrophic rhinitis. No toxigenic *Pasteurella multocida* type D has ever been isolated in regular monitoring from this herd and none is demonstrated in these pigs. A piglet is killed and the head split (*Figure 175*). The histological appearance of the nasal mucosa is seen in *Figure 176*. No *P. multocida* type D can be isolated.

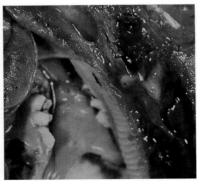

Figure 175

(a) What is the disease?
(b) What can be done about it?

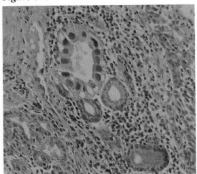

Figure 176

151 A similar outbreak of sneezing occurs in another high health herd and once again there is no evidence for the presence of toxigenic *Pasteurella multocida* type D. Progressive atrophic rhinitis does not develop although there is some degree of turbinate atrophy. Some affected piglets die and others have clearly developed pneumonia. When an animal is examined post-mortem the lungs appear as shown in *Figure 177*. What is your diagnosis and how would you treat and prevent the condition?

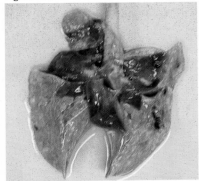

Figure 177

Sheep

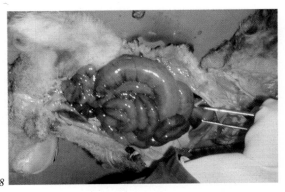

Figure 178

152 This 4-week-old lamb (*Figure 178*) on a restricted artificial feeding system was found dead a few hours after having appeared to be thriving normally. On opening the abdominal cavity, the intestines were seen to be dark red and distended with gas.
(a) What is the most likely cause of death?
(b) How may this be confirmed?
(c) What is the proposed aetiology of this condition?

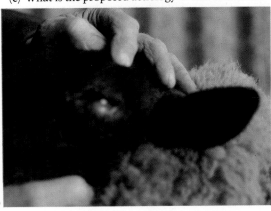

Figure 179

153 This sheep (*Figure 179*) was one of several in a flock showing bilateral ocular discharge and varying degrees of keratoconjunctivitis.
(a) What are the most likely causal agents?
(b) How is the disease spread?

Figure 180

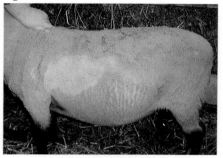

154 Wool loss (*Figure 180*) was seen in several ewes sheared after housing for the winter. Most of the loss occurred along the flanks of the animals and there were no signs of pruritis.
(a) What is your diagnosis?
(b) What is the proposed aetiology?

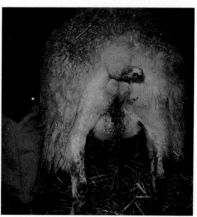

155 This ewe (*Figure 181*) has failed to expel the placenta after lambing.
(a) What is the incidence of this condition in sheep as compared with cattle?
(b) What are the possible causes?

Figure 181

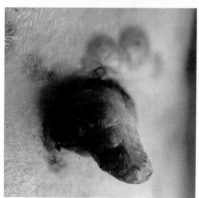

156 Vesicles are visible on the teats and udder of this ewe (*Figure 182*) which lambed 3 weeks previously.
(a) What is the likely cause?
(b) How may it be confirmed?
(c) What are the possible sequelae to this condition?

Figure 182

157 (a) What is the common name for this granulomatous condition (*Figure 183*) affecting the lower parts of the limbs in this animal?
(b) What are the organisms likely to be involved?

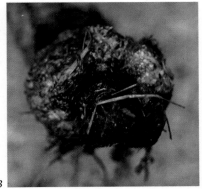

Figure 183

158 (a) What organisms are implicated in this common cause of lameness in sheep (*Figure 184*)?
(b) How is it commonly transmitted?
(c) What control measures are available?

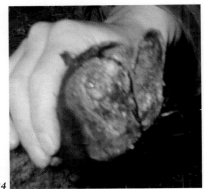

Figure 184

159 This 2-week-old lamb (*Figure 185*) was noticed to be walking stiffly the previous day. It is now rigid and unable to stand.
(a) What is the diagnosis?
(b) How can the disease be prevented?

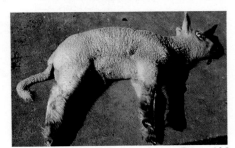

Figure 185

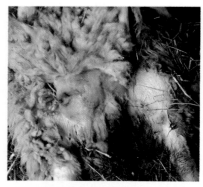

160 The udder of this lactating ewe (*Figure 186*) is purple and cold on one side.
(a) What is this condition?
(b) What are the common causal organisms?
(c) What are the common sequelae to this condition?

Figure 186

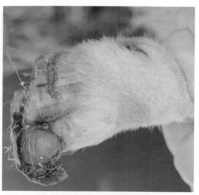

161 (a) What is this condition (*Figure 187*)?
(b) How does it commonly arise?
(c) How may it be successfully treated?

Figure 187

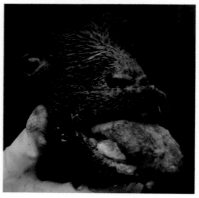

162 (a) What condition is affecting this 2-week-old lamb (*Figure 188*)?
(b) What are the likely sequelae?

Figure 188

163 This winter shorn sheep (*Figure 189*) was one of many in the group showing circular scabby lesions on the flanks.
(a) What is the diagnosis?
(b) How might infection have occurred?

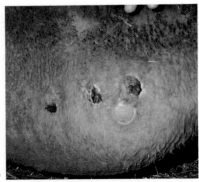

Figure 189

164 A large number of sheep in this flock showed lesions on the head, particularly around the eyes and nose (*Figure 190*). Affected areas became hairless and showed black scabs which bled when disturbed.
(a) What is the cause?
(b) What contributes to the spread of infection?

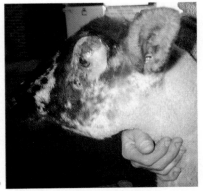

Figure 190

165 This ewe showed multiple discharging abscesses on the cheeks and jaw region (*Figure 191*).
(a) What are the possible diagnoses?
(b) What is the outcome?

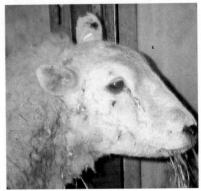

Figure 191

83

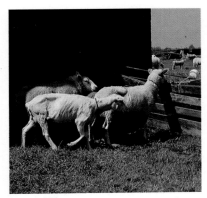

Figure 192

166 These sheep from a Dutch flock (*Figure 192*) were showing progressive weight loss and laboured respiration.
(a) What is the likely cause?
(b) How may it be diagnosed?
(c) What organs, other than the lungs, does this disease affect?
(d) How does the disease spread through the flock?

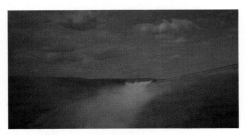

Figure 193

167 The grazing on this hill land (*Figure 193*) is being improved by ploughing and liming.
(a) What difference is this likely to make to the availability of trace elements to sheep grazing subsequently?
(b) What clinical conditions may result?

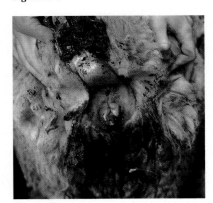

Figure 194

168 This ewe shows ulceration and swelling of the external genitalia (*Figure 194*).
(a) What organisms may be implicated?
(b) What are the common predisposing factors?

169 (a) What is this common condition (*Figure 195*)?
(b) What is the aetiology?

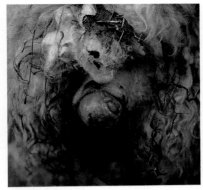

Figure 195

170 This fat ewe gave birth to a single lamb weighing only 2 kg (*Figure 196*). What were the likely events which led to this outcome?

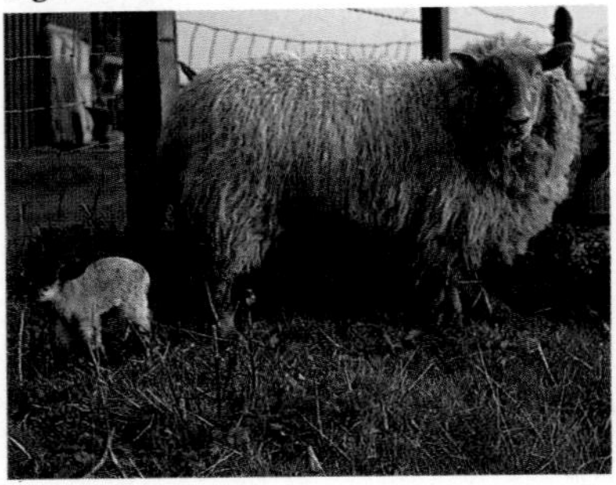

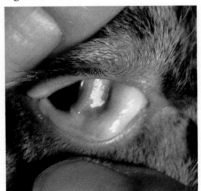

Figure 196

171 This 10-day-old lamb was lethargic and ceased feeding. Examination of the eye showed white mucous membranes (*Figure 197*).
(a) What essential question needs to be asked concerning the history of this lamb?
(b) What post-mortem finding would confirm the diagnosis?

Figure 197

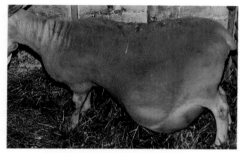

172 (a) What condition is affecting this pregnant ewe (*Figure 198*)?
(b) What is the likely cause?
(c) What is the likely outcome?

Figure 198

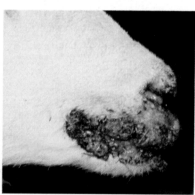

173 What is the common link between these two conditions (*Figure 199* and *200*)?

Figure 199

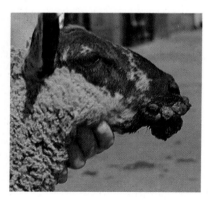

Figure 200

174 This Suffolk ram showed loss of weight and pruritis (*Figure 201*).
(a) What is the likely diagnosis?
(b) How may it be confirmed?
(c) What other signs may be seen in affected animals?

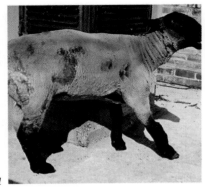

Figure 201

175 This yearling Welsh sheep was found with gross swelling of the head and ears and exudation around the eyes and mouth (*Figure 202*). What is the likely cause?

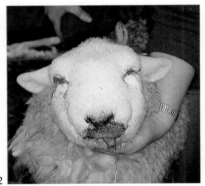

Figure 202

176 If no action is taken to assist the ewe (*Figure 203*) in the care of these newly born quadruplets, what is the most likely outcome?

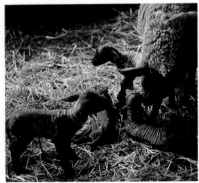

Figure 203

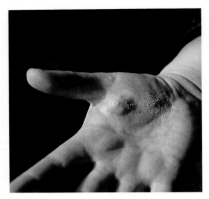

177 What is the possible cause of this painful lesion (*Figure 204*) which developed on the hand of a woman who was bottle-feeding young lambs?

Figure 204

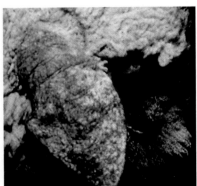

178 This animal showed numerous small scabs on the ears and face (*Figure 205*). No pruritis was evident.
(a) What is the probable diagnosis?
(b) How may it be confirmed?

Figure 205

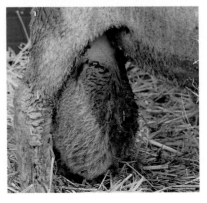

179 This ram showed gross enlargement of the scrotum (*Figure 206*). What are the possible diagnoses?

Figure 206

180 This 4-day-old lamb was scouring profusely (*Figure 207*).
(a) What are the common causes of scour in young lambs?
(b) How may they be differentiated?

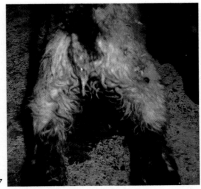

Figure 207

181 This 7-day-old lamb shows excess lachrymation and keratitis (*Figure 208*).
(a) What is the cause?
(b) Comment on treatment of the condition.

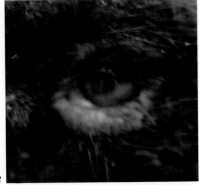

Figure 208

182 Comment on the appearance of the anal region of this 2-day-old lamb (*Figure 209*).

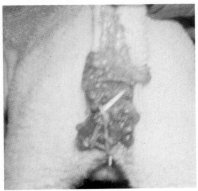

Figure 209

183 These 36-hour-old lambs (*Figure 210* and *211*) from the same flock both show wetness around the mouth. One lamb is collapsed with a distended abdomen (*Figure 211*).
(a) What is the condition?
(b) What is the proposed sequence of events leading to its onset?

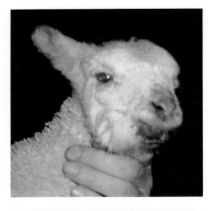

Figure 210

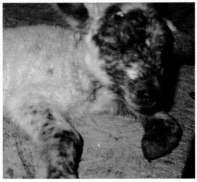

Figure 211

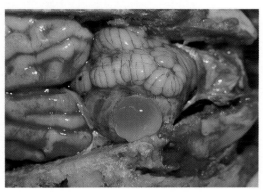

184 (a) What is this condition (*Figure 212*)?
(b) What clinical signs would you expect to see associated with the lesion in this site?

Figure 212

185 This 2-year-old Welsh ram (*Figure 213*) shows unilateral paralysis of the muscles of the cheek, mouth and ear, with intense depression.
(a) What is the likely diagnosis?
(b) How may it be confirmed?
(c) What particular management features are associated with the condition?
(d) How does infection gain entry into the body?

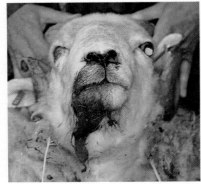

Figure 213

186 These intestines (*Figure 214*) came from a sheep which showed progressive loss of condition over several months.
(a) What chronic bacterial infection could be involved?
(b) How may diagnosis be confirmed?
(c) Can this disease be diagnosed in the live animal?

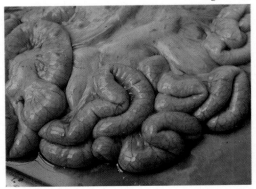

Figure 214

187 These lungs (*Figure 215*) are heavier than normal and the lower portions show well demarcated solid grey areas.
(a) What is the likely diagnosis?
(b) What characteristic feature would be seen in an affected live animal?
(c) What infectious agents are associated with this condition?

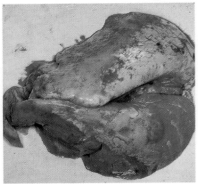

Figure 215

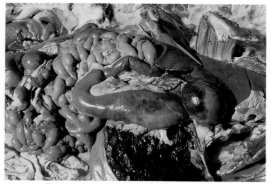

188 This hogg was found dead in late autumn. Postmortem examination showed acute inflammation of the abomasum (*Figure 216*).
(a) What is the likely cause of death?
(b) How may it be prevented?

Figure 216

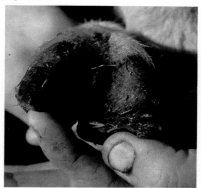

189 This ram shows an out-growth of skin in the interdigital space (*Figure 217*).
(a) What is the common name of the feature?
(b) What advice should the owner be given?

Figure 217

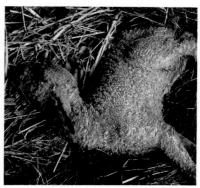

190 This lamb (*Figure 218*) was one of six which were unable to stand after birth and showed severe opisthotonus.
(a) What is the name of this condition?
(b) What advice should be given to the owner of these pedigree sheep?

Figure 218

191 Comment on the health status during the past few months of the animal from which this wool sample was taken (*Figure 219*).

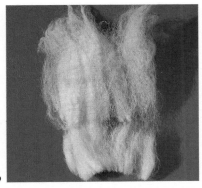

Figure 219

192 This yearling female (*Figure 220*) was from a flock of prolific Milksheep, in which a significant number of maiden ewes failed to breed. Comment on the breeding potential of this animal.

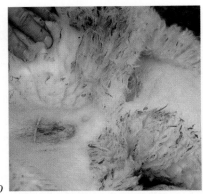

Figure 220

193 At a routine culling examination in early Autumn, several ewes were noticed to have areas of wool loss with scab formation on the back or hindquarters (*Figure 221*). The lesions were not pruritic at this stage. What was the likely cause?

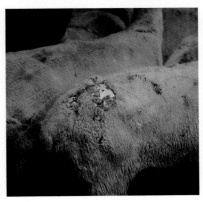

Figure 221

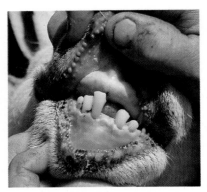

194   Comment on the incisor teeth of this ram (*Figure 222*).

Figure 222

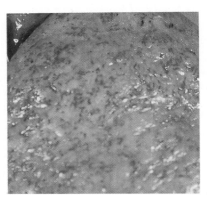

195   What events have led up to the appearance of the udder of this ewe (*Figure 223*)?

Figure 223

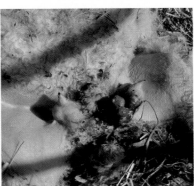

196   Six ewe-lambs out of a flock of 150 are found dead one morning in December; several of the remainder are very reluctant to move. The livers of the dead lambs all show lesions as illustrated in *Figure 224*.
(a) What is the diagnosis?
(b) What advice would you give?

Figure 224

197 Three ewes aborted on one day and this is one of the placentas (*Figure 225*).
(a) Describe the lesions and indicate the diagnosis.
(b) How would you confirm the diagnosis?

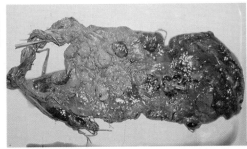

Figure 225

198 This 4-week-old Swaledale lamb (*Figure 226*) has developed a severe arthritis in a number of joints, particularly the carpal and tarsal joints. What is the most likely cause?

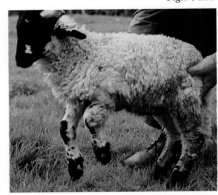

Figure 226

199 This foetus (*Figure 227*) was produced with a live weak lamb by a ewe-lamb a few days before the expected lambing date.
(a) What do you think was responsible?
(b) How could you confirm your diagnosis?

Figure 227

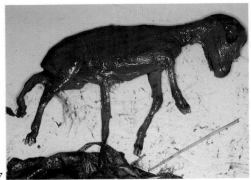

Figure 228

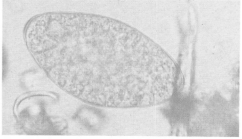

200 These eggs (*Figure 228*), which measure 140 × 75 μm were found in the faeces of a 3-year-old ewe which had a condition score of 1.5.
(a) What is your diagnosis?
(b) What would you do with this ewe and the rest of the flock?

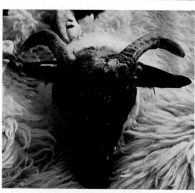

201 (a) What is the cause of these wounds around the horns (*Figure 229*) of these Scottish Blackface sheep?
(b) What steps would you take to reduce the incidence next year?

Figure 229

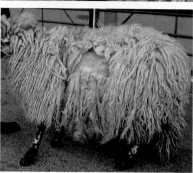

Figure 230

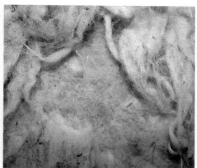

Figure 231

202 These two photographs (*Figure 230* and *231*) are of a Swaledale hogg in Winter.
(a) What is the most likely cause of the pruritic lesions?
(b) How would you confirm your diagnosis?
(c) What treatment would you recommend?

203 (a) What information can you obtain from the straw attached to the hindleg of this ram (*Figure 232*)?
(b) What further examination would you carry out?

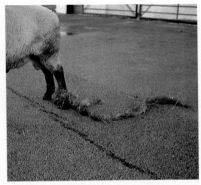

Figure 232

204 This 4-year-old ewe (*Figure 233*) had a condition score of 1 and was one of three similar ewes in a flock of 200.
(a) What are the possible causes?
(b) How would you attempt to arrive at a specific diagnosis?

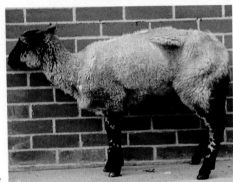

Figure 233

205 Comment on the appearance of the foot of this sheep (*Figure 234*).

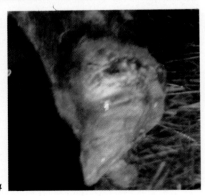

Figure 234

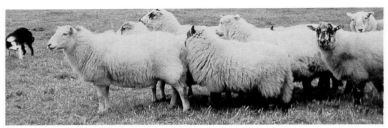

Figure 235

206 Sheepdogs (Border collies) are essential to sheep farming (*Figure 235*), especially in hill areas but they may be responsible for disease in the sheep.
(a) What are the most important conditions in sheep which may be transmitted from dogs?
(b) What steps would you recommend to reduce the risks?

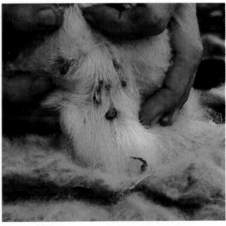

Figure 236

207 These ectoparasites were found on a high proportion of the Swaledale lambs (*Figure 236*) in a flock in North Yorkshire.
(a) What are they?
(b) What is their importance?
(c) What control measures are available for them and the diseases they transmit?

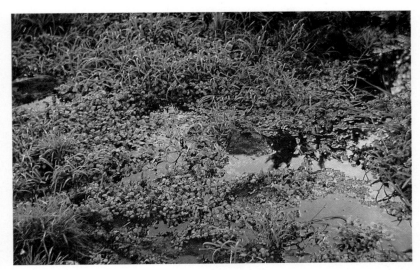

Figure 237

208 A 44-year-old man had a caravan in the English Lake District and frequently ate this plant (*Figure 237*) from a very wet area near the caravan site. He spent his summer holiday at the site and the following Christmas developed abdominal pain, vomiting, nausea and jaundice. What advice would you give to his doctor, who thinks that he may have caught something from the animals on the farm near the site?

209 This 4-year-old ewe (*Figure 238*) has been losing condition over the last few months, has been coughing and shows respiratory distress when gathered for vaccination. She is now passing fluid from her nostrils.
(a) What is the most likely diagnosis?
(b) How could it be confirmed?
(c) Is serology useful?
(d) What advice would you give in order to control the condition?

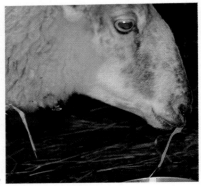

Figure 238

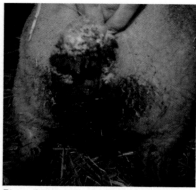

Figure 239

210 This 8-week-old lamb (*Figure 239*) has been in a small field since it was turned out 6 weeks ago.
(a) What are the most likely causes of the profuse scouring?
(b) How would you confirm your diagnosis?
(c) What would you do to treat the lamb?

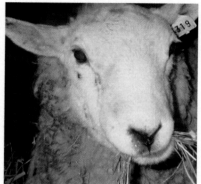

Figure 240

211 What are the most likely reasons for this ewe (*Figure 240*) having hay protruding from its mouth almost continuously?

Poultry

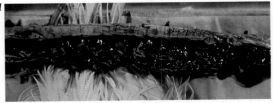

Figure 241

212 This acute intestinal problem (*Figure 241*) causes mortality in chickens of all ages over 3 weeks of age. The condition can affect up to 100% of the flock. Affected birds are disinclined to come to the feed.
(a) What is the name and cause of this condition?
(b) Is this seen as an individual bird problem or a flock problem?
(c) How would one treat this condition?
(d) How can the condition be prevented in broilers and replacement layers?
(e) What management factors will increase the incidence of the condition?

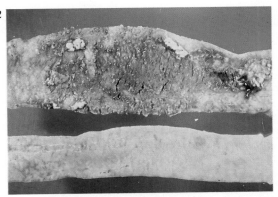

Figure 242

213 This intestinal condition (*Figure 242*) is seen mainly in young birds, although it has been seen in adults, and is usually restricted to a small percentage of the flock.
(a) What is the cause of this condition?
(b) Where does the causal agent normally reside in the bird?
(c) What is a differential diagnosis?
(d) What would be the treatment?
(e) What is the expected mortality likely to be in untreated cases?

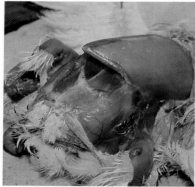

Figure 243

214 A continuing mortality seen in good birds within a broiler flock, this condition (*Figure 243*) is seen more during the winter than the summer.
(a) What is the condition?
(b) What are the suspected causes?
(c) What age does it usually appear?
(d) Is any treatment or preventative measure possible?

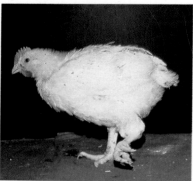

Figure 244

215 This is a type of leg weakness in broilers (*Figure 244*).
(a) What is this condition called and is it a common problem?
(b) What is the cause?
(c) How can the incidence of this condition be influenced?
(d) What other conditions affect the bones of broilers causing leg weakness in the flock?

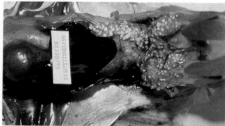

Figure 245

216 This respiratory condition (*Figure 245*) is seen in all species of domestic poultry, wild birds and zoo collections.

(a) What is the name and cause of this condition?
(b) What other organs may show lesions?
(c) How is the disease transmitted?
(d) At what age are chickens, turkeys and ducks most susceptible?
(e) What is the differential diagnosis to be considered when only lung lesions are present?
(f) How would one deal with an outbreak?

Figure 246

217 This common condition (*Figure 246*) is found in broilers and in other types of domestic birds.

(a) What is this condition?

(b) Can it be confused with any other condition?

(c) What are the predisposing factors precipitating this disease?

(d) If the condition was seen on the processing line in the slaughter house, what would be the action of the Official Veterinary Surgeon?

(e) What is the main route of entry for the causal agent in birds?

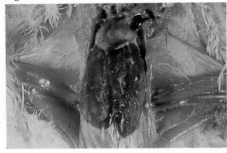

(f) How would the flock be treated?

218 This condition is sometimes seen when carrying out a postmortem (*Figure 247*) on young chickens, poults and ducklings. The caeca are full of necrotic cores.

(a) What is this condition?

(b) What is the differential diagnosis?

(c) How is the diagnosis confirmed?

(d) What other lesions might one find in such diseased birds?

(e) How would the infection have been transmitted?

(f) What would be the effect of treatment?

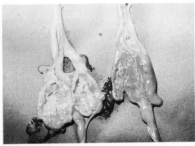

Figure 247

219 This condition (*Figure 248*) is a common cause of sudden mortality in adolescent and older turkeys.

(a) What is this condition?

(b) What are the other causes of sudden death in turkeys?

(c) Is there any treatment that would be successful?

(d) What advice would you give the farmer?

(e) What is the appearance of the carcase?

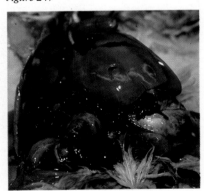

Figure 248

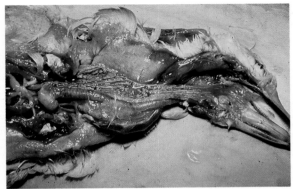

Figure 249

220 This condition commonly affects adult ducks (*Figure 249*) on open pond systems.
(a) What is this condition?
(b) What are the common post-mortem findings?
(c) How is the diagnosis confirmed?
(d) Can it be confused with any other condition?
(e) How is the condition introduced into a flock?
(f) Is there any treatment?

Figure 250

221 (a) What is this condition (*Figure 250*) of commercial ducks?
(b) What age group are commonly affected?
(c) What are the typical clinical signs?
(d) How can the disease be treated/controlled?

222 (a) What is this condition (*Figure 251*) of commercial ducks?
(b) What are the typical clinical signs?
(c) How is the disease confirmed?
(d) What diseases should be considered in differential diagnosis?
(e) Is there any effective treatment?
(f) What are the predisposing factors?

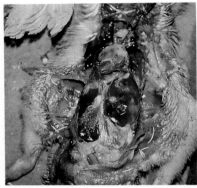

Figure 251

223 The poultry meat inspector at a broiler plant presents you with several carcases with this generalised skin lesion (*Figure 252*).
(a) What is this condition?
(b) How is it caused?
(c) How can the problem be rectified?
(d) What would your judgement be with respect to the carcase fitness for human consumption?

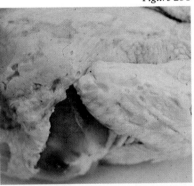

Figure 252

224 At meat inspection, a flock of broilers being processed shows a large percentage of birds with black scabby lesions affecting the backs of the hocks (*Figure 253*).
(a) What is this condition?
(b) What other parts of the carcase are often affected?
(c) What is the cause of this problem?
(d) What action will be required at meat inspection?

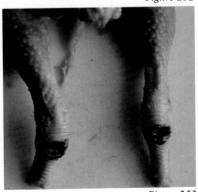

Figure 253

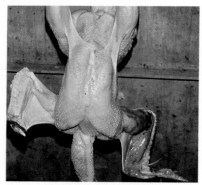

Figure 254

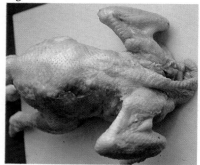

Figure 255

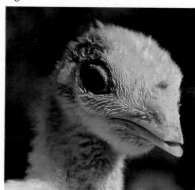

Figure 256

225 A high incidence of this type of lesion (*Figure 254*) is detected on whole body inspection of a batch of fattening turkeys on a processing line.
(a) What is the cause of this condition and what accounts for the distinct colour change?
(b) When would it have occurred and how old are the lesions?
(c) What action would be required at meat inspection?

226 Several birds have been rejected as unfit for human consumption from a broiler processing line with green lesions over the back. *Figure 255* shows a typical case.
(a) What is the cause of this staining?
(b) What are the possible risks to human health from such a carcase?
(c) Should the carcases have been rejected as unfit?
(d) What steps could be taken to reduce the incidence of this condition in the plant?

227 A group of 3-week-old turkeys show a sudden onset of lethargy, snicking, mouth breathing, coughing, foamy ocular discharge and sticky nasal discharge affecting nearly 100% of the birds (*Figure 256*). Several days later, more severe sinus swelling and submandibular oedema is seen and several poults die.
(a) What is this condition?
(b) What is the causal agent?
(c) What proportion of birds are likely to die?
(d) What factors affect mortality?

(e) What other avian species are affected by this agent?
(f) What control measures are available?

228 Several broiler breeder pullets are found in a laying flock, sitting in this typical posture (*Figure 257*).
(a) What is this condition?
(b) What is likely to be the extent of the problem in a flock and are there any effects on production?
(c) What are the typical lesions at post-mortem?
(d) Has a cause for this condition been established and is there any treatment?

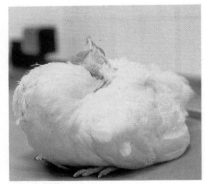

Figure 257

229 A group of free range layers becomes affected by scabby lesions of the face, combs and wattles (*Figure 258*).
(a) What is this condition?
(b) What other avian species may be affected?
(c) Where else may lesions be detected?
(d) Which conditions need to be considered in differential diagnosis?
(e) How could a diagnosis be confirmed?
(f) How can the condition be controlled?

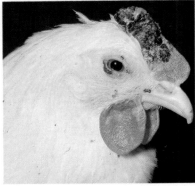

Figure 258

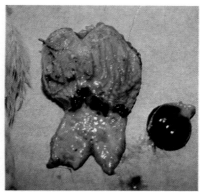

Figure 259

(a) What is this acute viral disease and what other avian species may be affected?
(b) What other typical lesions can be detected at post-mortem?
(c) How can a diagnosis be confirmed?
(d) What are the likely sequelae in an infected flock?
(e) How can the disease be controlled?
(f) When presented with post-mortem lesions as in *Figure 259*, what other important virus disease of poultry needs to be considered in a differential diagnosis?

230 Sudden high mortality occurs in a flock of commercial broiler chickens. Amongst the post-mortem lesions are striking haemorrhages in the bursa of fabricius and at the proventricular/gizzard junction (*Figure 259*).

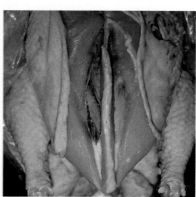

Figure 260

231 This lesion (*Figure 260*) is detected sporadically in broiler and turkey cutting plants and very occasionally by the housewife at the table in the roasted bird.
(a) What is the name of this condition?
(b) Which muscle is affected?
(c) What is the cause of this condition?
(d) What is the public health significance of this lesion?

232 Several free range hens in a small, recently set up, backyard system are reported to be losing condition, in spite of regular worming. One bird dies and post-mortem reveals the lesions shown in the intestines (*Figure 261*).
(a) What is this condition?
(b) What are the causes of this condition and how can it be prevented?

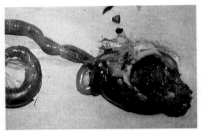

Figure 261

233 A group of fattening turkeys shows sudden onset sinus swelling (*Figure 262*), sneezing, rales and mouth breathing. Many of the birds are seen to wipe their faces against the leading edge of their wings.
(a) What is this condition?
(b) How can a clinical diagnosis be confirmed?
(c) How can a flock become infected?
(d) How can the disease be controlled?

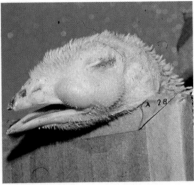

Figure 262

234 A high proportion of 2-week-old broiler chicks show bizarre nervous signs (*Figure 263*) such as weakness, ataxia, violent spasmodic inco-ordination, torticollis and death.
(a) What is this condition?
(b) What virtually pathognomic lesions are detected at post-mortem?
(c) What conditions need to be considered in a differential diagnosis?
(d) How can the condition be treated and prevented?

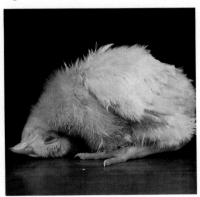

Figure 263

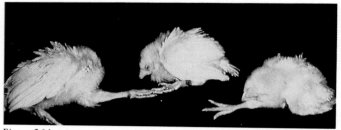

Figure 264

235 A high proportion of 2-week-old broiler chicks show ataxia, fine tremors and a tendency to sit down on their hocks (*Figure 264*). Birds progress to paralysis and death.
(a) What is this condition?
(b) How can the condition be diagnosed?
(c) How do chicks become infected?
(d) What factors affect morbidity rate?
(e) What signs are seen in laying breeder flocks?

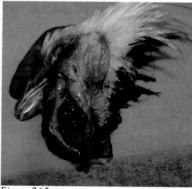

Figure 265

236 5% of a flock of broiler breeders shows depression, dirty eyes and conjunctivitis with swelling of the wattles as illustrated (*Figure 265*).
(a) What is this condition and how can this be confirmed?
(b) What other post-mortem lesions can be seen?
(c) What are the possible sources of infection?
(d) What control or treatment measures are available?

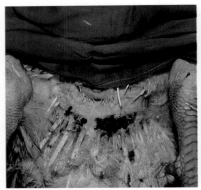

Figure 266

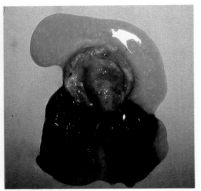

Figure 267

237 There have been several recent deaths in fattening turkeys and others are noted with black, scabby lesions around the vent, tail and legs (*Figure 266*).
(a) What is the likely cause of these lesions?
(b) What other problems may be precipitated?

238 This lesion is detected in a proportion of broiler chickens at meat inspection. The affected pericardial sac contains either floccular fluid or more purulent viscous material (*Figure 267*). A proportion of other birds show severe polyserositis, poor colour and uneveness.
(a) What is the cause of this lesion?
(b) What other conditions could it be confused with?
(c) What clinical picture is likely to have occurred during the life of the broiler crop?

239 Sporadically, several broiler chickens have shown this type of characteristic posture (*Figure 268*) between 4 and 6 weeks of age. The affected birds sit back on their hocks and tend to topple backwards with one or both feet off the ground and wings held out for balance.
(a) What is this condition?
(b) What is the cause?
(c) With what other conditions may it be confused?

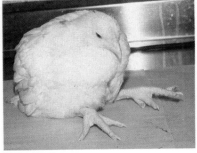

Figure 268

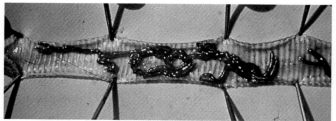
Figure 269

240 A group of 6-week-old pheasants show repetitive mouth opening, pronounced respiratory effort and neck stretching. A few birds have blood present in the mouth. There have been several recent sudden deaths (*Figure 269*).
(a) What is this condition?
(b) List the important aspects of the life-cycle of the causal agent.
(c) How would you treat an infected group?

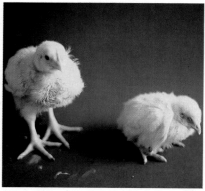
Figure 270

241 A large number of 3-week-old broilers appear weak, pale and stunted (*Figure 270*). Only 2 houses out of 6 on the site appear affected. Many have wet and haemorrhagic lesions at the wing tips. At post-mortem, the bursa, thymus and spleen appear atrophied.
(a) What is the causal agent of this condition?
(b) How do chicks become infected and why were only 2 houses affected?

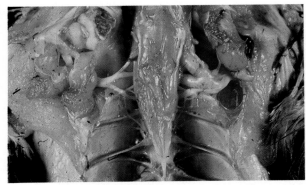

242 A flock of free-range pullets recently placed on a site at 16 weeks of age experience an increase in mortality and some fairly ill-defined nervous signs such as wing droop and some lameness. Pullets are pale and somewhat under target weight. Post-mortem examination reveals few lesions in 3 culled birds other than unilateral swelling of the brachial nerve plexus (*Figure 271*) and a thickened sciatic nerve.
(a) What is this condition and how can the diagnosis be confirmed?
(b) What is the likely outcome for the flock?
(c) What factors may account for apparent vaccination failures?

Figure 272

243 A turkey breeder suspects his flock has been poisoned. Several dead hens are found with others appearing dull, lethargic and reluctant to stand. The following day many more have died. Affected birds show dark crusty lesions notably affecting the head (*Figure 272*). At post-mortem there are widespread petechial haemorrhages in fat, skin and muscles. The liver is enlarged and congested and, in some birds, has a cooked appearance.
(a) What is the condition and how would you confirm this?
(b) What is the likely source of infection?

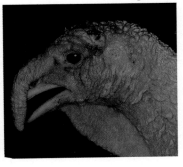

(c) How can the disease be controlled?
(d) What is the public health significance of this condition?

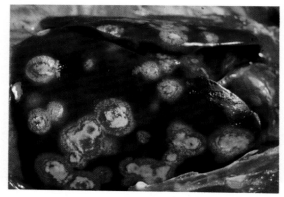

Figure 273

244 An arable farmer fattens a group of turkeys for the Christmas trade in a converted barn with straw yard and extensive earth run. The group as a whole fail to thrive, some passing yellow unpleasant droppings. One bird dies and is submitted for post-mortem examination and shows these striking liver lesions (*Figure 273*).
(a) What is this condition?
(b) What other organ is also seriously affected?
(c) Name the nematode worm important in the spread of this condition and explain the significance of the earthworm in its epidemiology.
(d) What control measures are available?

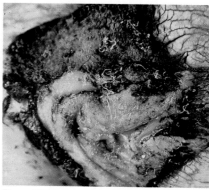

Figure 274

245 A group of 5-week-old free-range goslings are suspected by the owner to have been poisoned. Most of the birds are very dopey and several are reluctant to stand, appearing to be lame (*Figure 274*).
(a) What is the cause of this condition?
(b) What lesions would you expect to see at post-mortem and how does this relate to the lameness reported?
(c) How can the condition be treated?

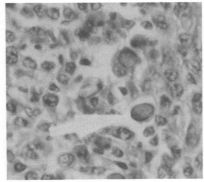

Figure 275

246 A flock of commercial fattening turkeys experience sudden onset of dark tarry droppings, with several sudden deaths. At post-mortem, the intestinal contents are blood-stained and the spleen enlarged and mottled. The affected spleen shows these histological changes (*Figure 275*).
(a) What is this condition?
(b) What significant histological changes are demonstrated above?
(c) What other tests may be used to confirm a diagnosis?
(d) What factors can precipitate an outbreak and is there any specific treatment?
(e) The causal agent is known to affect two other avian species. Which are they and what are the clinical and pathological results of such infection?

Figure 276

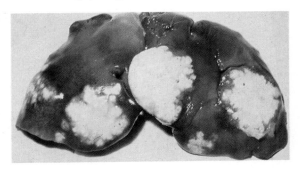

247 Several turkeys on the processing line show these distinct liver lesions (*Figure 276*).
(a) What is the name of this condition?
(b) How does it arise?
(c) What is the clinical significance of this condition?

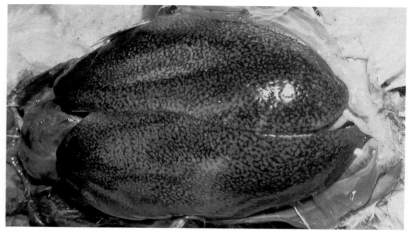

Figure 277

248 A broiler breeder flock is not performing to expected targets. There have been several recent deaths. One such bird shows this striking liver pathology (*Figure 277*).
(a) What is this condition?
(b) What other conditions must be considered in differential diagnosis?
(c) How can a diagnosis be confirmed?
(d) What control measures are available?

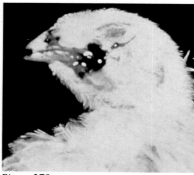

Figure 278

249 On a multiage laying site, some of the youngest point of lay pullets exhibit severe respiratory signs with gasping, moist rales, coughing, nasal discharge and conjunctivitis. Several birds show blood clots at the mouth and nares (*Figure 278*).
(a) What is this condition?
(b) What is the likely effect on older birds on the site?
(c) How can the disease be confirmed?
(d) How can the disease be controlled?

Figure 279

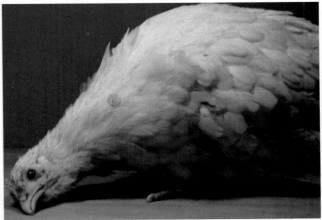

250 Several birds in a group of 12-week-old broiler breeder pullets show this typical posture (*Figure 279*). When removed to a hospital pen, affected birds recover within 1 or 2 days.
(a) What is this condition?
(b) What is the causal agent?
(c) What lesions will be seen at post-mortem?

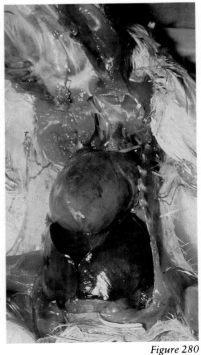

251 Eight 3-week-old turkey breeder poults in rear die suddenly. At post-mortem, this striking heart abnormality is detected (*Figure 280*).
(a) What is this condition?
(b) What is its cause?
(c) What histological features are detected in the liver?
(d) What is the typical pattern of mortality?

Figure 280

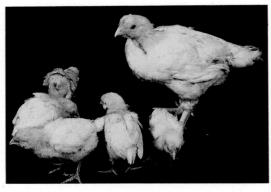

Figure 281

252 These 4-week-old broiler chickens are from a site where culling for uneveness has been excessive since birds were about 2 weeks old. About 10% of the 4-week-old birds still retain downy feathering of the head and back. Developing primary wing feathers have a very tatty appearance (*Figure 281*).
(a) What is this condition?
(b) What is its cause and what factors influence its severity?
(c) What lesions would be detectable at post-mortem at this age?

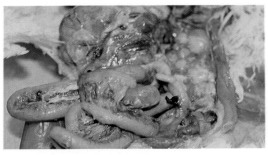

Figure 282

253 There is an increase in mortality in 24-week-old broiler breeder pullets coming into lay early and well. Six birds are presented for examination and all show the presence of inspissated yolk material throughout the abdomen (*Figure 282*) with resulting inflammation.
(a) What is this condition?
(b) What factors contribute to its incidence?
(c) Why is it always prudent to undertake bacteriological examinations in these outbreaks?

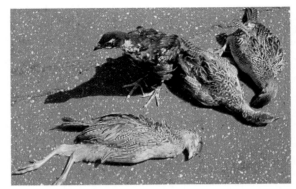

Figure 283

254 A group of pheasants in a release pen are found either dull, recumbent or dead (*Figure 283*). Some are obviously paralysed.
(a) What is this condition?
(b) How are the birds likely to have become affected?
(c) What other conditions should be considered in a differential diagnosis?

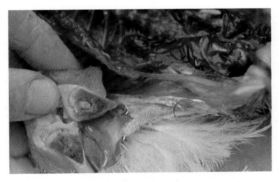

Figure 284

255 A group of 4-week-old broilers which were growing well show a number of acute and severely lame birds. At post-mortem there is little to see in the muscles or joints. However, sectioning of the long bones reveals these small lesions in the metaphyses of the long bones (*Figure 284*).
(a) What is this condition?
(b) What organisms are commonly involved?
(c) How may the condition arise?
(d) At what other sites may similar lesions develop and under what conditions?

Figure 285

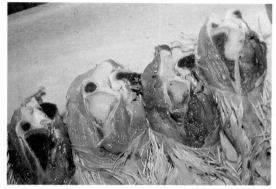

256 A flock of broiler chickens has been growing well but in the 6th week of life, a variety of leg problems have developed. A proportion show deformity of the tibia. When the proximal end of the tibia is sectioned, these lesions are easily visible (*Figure 285*).
(a) What is this condition?
(b) What is the cause of this lesion?
(c) What are the possible sequelae?

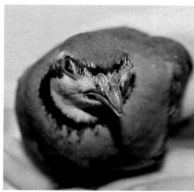

257 There are a number of sudden deaths in 5-week-old red-legged partridge in a large rearing pen. Others show a lethargy, drooping wings and signs of 'head cold' such as mouth breathing, conjunctivitis and nasal discharge (*Figure 286*).
(a) What is this condition?
(b) What lesions are seen at post-mortem?
(c) What advice would you give for treatment and control?

Figure 286

Figure 287

258 At the height of a full racing season, a novice pigeon keeper complains that several of his birds have leg swellings, especially around their rings (*Figure 287*), with a generalised scurfy appearance to the legs and feet of several other birds.
(a) What is this condition?
(b) What is its cause?
(c) How can the condition be treated?

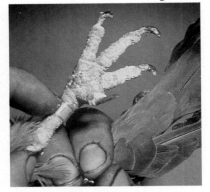

259 Several pigeons from a racing loft show blepharospasm, conjunctivitis and slight nasal discharge (*Figure 288*).
(a) What is the common name for this condition?
(b) What are its causes?
(c) How can the condition be treated?

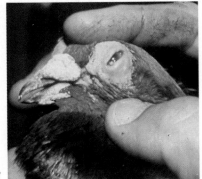

Figure 288

260 A large number of broiler breeders show obvious head flicking, slight snick, blepharospasm, mild ocular discharge and corneal opacity (*Figure 289*).
(a) What is this condition?
(b) What are the likely causes?
(c) What other sequelae may follow?

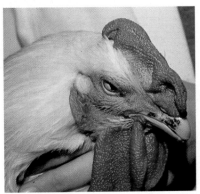

Figure 289

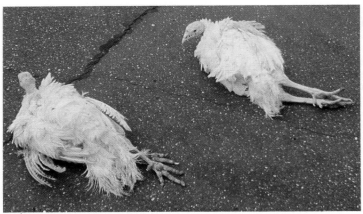

Figure 290

261 A group of 10-week-old turkeys experiences the severe respiratory disease associated with *Mycoplasma gallisepticum* infection. Treatment with tiamulin is instigated and respiratory signs rapidly subside. However, at the same time, birds become drowsy, their wings droop and many show flaccid paralysis of the legs (*Figure 290*).
(a) What is the cause of this apparent toxicity?
(b) What lesions are seen at post-mortem?
(c) How can a diagnosis be confirmed?

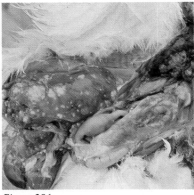

Figure 291

262 A client has a small breeding flock of silkie bantams. It is noticed that several birds have become lethargic and there is obvious loss of weight, in spite of continued good appetite. One such bird dies suddenly and shows extensive lesions as illustrated (*Figure 291*).
(a) What is this condition?
(b) Which organs are commonly affected?
(c) How can a diagnosis be confirmed?
(d) How can the condition be controlled in a small valuable breeding collection?

263 A broiler breeder flock exhibits sudden loss of egg numbers and shell colour a few days after a feed delivery (*Figure 292*). Over the next few days, egg size is also adversely affected.
(a) What is the cause of this problem?
(b) How could this have arisen?
(c) What are the likely sequelae to the problem?

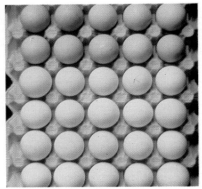

Figure 292

264 Which of the following diseases is caused by a herpes virus?
(a) Infectious laryngotracheitis.
(b) Duck virus hepatitis type 1.
(c) Infectious bursal disease.
(d) Marek's disease.
(e) Duck virus enteritis.
(f) Lymphoid leukosis.

265 To which virus genus do the causal agents of the following diseases belong?
(a) Egg drop syndrome '76.
(b) Duck virus hepatitis type 2.
(c) Infectious bursal disease.
(d) Newcastle disease.
(e) Infectious bronchitis.
(f) Avian influenza (fowl plague).
(g) Epidemic tremor.
(h) Turkey rhinotracheitis.

266 This type of lesion was detected in a flock of free-range laying hens affecting the feet (*Figure 293*) and shanks of several birds.
(a) What is this condition?
(b) What is its cause?
(c) With what other diseases may this problem be confused?

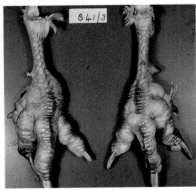

Figure 293

267 A broiler producer complains of high first week mortality in his intake of chicks. List 5 possible diagnoses on post-mortem examination.

268 Name 5 zoonotic disease agents transmissible to man from avian species.

269 Cross contamination within a poultry processing operation can result in significant bacterial contamination of otherwise clean carcases.
(a) List 8 main areas where this can occur.
(b) Indicate the 2 most important areas.

270 Indicate the welfare problems that may arise during the collection and processing of broilers.

271 Broiler breeders may be fed on a single sex feeding system.
(a) What is this technique?
(b) Why is it necessary?
(c) How is the male prevented from eating the females' food?

272 What are the main points to look for in the brooding of young birds?

273 Probiotics have been advocated for use in poultry diets.
(a) What are they?
(b) What are their suggested beneficial effects?
(c) What are their suggested modes of action?

274 What are the possible methods used throughout the production process to reduce the risk of contamination of finished poultry feeds with salmonella?

275 Clostridia are ubiquitous Gram-positive bacteria, frequently found in the birds' environment and in low numbers in the normal bird's intestinal tract.
(a) List 3 diseases associated with clostridia in poultry, and the bacterial species involved in each case.
(b) How do birds become infected and what predisposing factors are important in each disease?
(c) How can each of the conditions be controlled?

ANSWERS

Cattle

1 (a) A popliteal abscess, caused by a septic focus (e.g. white-line infection) in the lower limb.
(b) The popliteal lymph node is situated deep in the quadriceps muscle mass and abscesses frequently need to be left for 2–3 months before they become sufficiently superficial to be lanced and drained. Repeated flushing with warm antiseptic solutions every second day for 1–2 weeks assists resolution.

2 (a) Malignant Catarrhal Fever (MCF).
(b) The genome of the MCF virus is thought to become incorporated into the genetic material of the large granular lymphocytes. These lymphocytes then lose their ability to control T-lymphocytes and, at the same time, they begin an autodestruction of mucosal surfaces. The virus is carried by sheep, wildebeest and possibly deer.
(c) MCF is invariably fatal and affected animals should be culled as soon as the diagnosis has been made.

3 (a) An epiphyseal fracture and partial dislocation.
(b) Very poor. Epiphyseal fractures do not heal well. (The prognosis for a metaphyseal fracture in a calf of this age is very good.) In addition, the open discharging wound on the lateral carpus indicates secondary infection.

4 (a) Nutritional enteropathy, coccidiosis, cryptospiridiasis, chronic salmonellosis (unlikely with no pyrexia).
(b) Poor concentrate intakes preweaning, due to inadequate access, suboptimal palatability or high intakes of liquid feed. Unsuitable concentrate, e.g. high-starch products leading to ruminal acidosis, ulceration and poor development of ruminal papillae; indigestible and/or allergenic vegetable proteins. Acidic feedstuffs (e.g. silage or maize gluten) fed at high levels before the rumen is fully developed (i.e. less than 12–14 weeks old). Inadequate access to palatable forage.

5 (a) Spastic paresis ('Elso heel') and dorsal patellar luxation.
(b) Dorsal patellar luxation tends to produce a longer period of limb overextension, during which it may be possible to palpate the displaced patella. However, confirmation of the diagnosis may require response to medial patellar desmotomy.
(c) Tibial neurectomy can be performed, but it may not be easy to locate the tibial nerve. Section of the gastrocnemius tendon proximal to the hock is simple and effective. Although there is initial extreme hock flexion, this is soon counteracted and affected animals normally reach slaughter weight uneventfully. As it can be heritable, affected animals should not be bred.

6 (a) Bovine Viral Diarrhoea (BVD).
(b) In early pregnancy. Exposure of a non-immune dam to BVD virus in early/mid pregnancy often produces only a mild transient illness in the dam, but the virus can pass the placenta to become established in the foetus. If this occurs before the age of foetal immunological competence, then the foetus will continue to carry the virus for the rest of its life. The majority of such animals become infected with a more severe strain of BVD at between 3 and 24 months of age and develop the clinical syndrome of acute mucosal disease, which is invariably fatal.

(c) Serological testing would show that the affected heifer was BVD antigen positive but antibody negative.

7 (a) Joint ill.

(b) *A. pyogenes, E. coli* and streptococci. Predisposing factors include inadequate colostrum intake (poor/mismothering, prolonged parturition, dystocia, maternal illness), navel infections (failure to spray/dip navel, overcrowding/poor hygiene in calving boxes) and other conditions leading to pyaemia.

(c) Treatment depends on the severity of the condition. Intense parenteral antibiotic therapy (e.g. lincomycin at 10mg/kg daily for 10–15 days) possibly combined with anti-inflammatory agents, will resolve mild cases. Advanced infections may require flushing and drainage of the joint, but prognosis is then guarded. Polyarthritis cases, with multiple joint involvement, are best culled.

8 (a) Actinobacillosis ('wooden tongue'), caused by *Actinobacillus lignieresi*.

(b) Actinobacillosis lesions may also occur in the nostrils, producing restricted, roaring breathing; as large granulomatous lesions on the skin; and occasionally at the base of the oesophagus or in the oesophageal groove, where they may interfere with erructation to produce chronic bloat.

(c) *Actinobacillus* will respond to streptomycin and other antibiotics effective against gram-negative organisms. Prolonged therapy (7–14 days) may be required.

9 (a) Sunburn. As the lesions were totally confined to the left side of the teat, it is probable that the cow allowed excessive exposure of her left side to the sun.

(b) Licking eczema, or summer sores. This is thought to be due to a combination of fly irritation and damage from sunlight producing a moist, wet eczema at the base of the teat, sometimes extending onto the udder. Very occasionally lesions may also be seen on the skin of the flanks and navel.

(c) Prevent further exposure to sunlight. Apply the milking machine for the minimum possible time, even if this means not fully emptying the udder. Apply an emollient cream to the teats after each milking.

10 (a) Winter dysentery (winter diarrhoea). The aetiology is uncertain, although coronavirus has been implicated.

(b) i) Salmonellosis: usually a more severe illness involving a dysenteric diarrhoea and some mortality. Confirm by culture.

ii) Overeating, producing acidosis and rumenitis: it is most probable that all cows would have been exposed to the same common source of feedstuffs and hence all cases would occur at the same time. Particles of the engorged feed (e.g. maize, barley or fodder beet) may be visible in the faeces.

(c) Non-specific anti-scour therapy, e.g. kaolin and astringents. Many cases recover spontaneously.

11 (a) Cerebrocortical necrosis, CCN, also known as polioencephalomalacia. Meningitis and poisoning, e.g. with lead, would be the main differentials. Meningitis cases are generally pyrexic. Lead poisoning should give a history of access.

(b) CCN is an induced thiamine deficiency, produced by proliferation of the ruminal thiaminase-producing bacteria *Bacillus thiaminolyticus* and *Clostridium sporogenes*.

Disease is most common on high concentrate/low-fibre diets which both favour the growth of the organisms and increase the ruminal requirement for thiamine. Outbreaks can be associated with digestive upsets.

(c) Even quite advanced nervous signs respond to high doses of parenteral thiamine, provided that it is given early in the course of the disease.

12 (a) Winter (type II) ostertagiasis.

(b) In the live animal, serum pepsinogen levels will be elevated due to abomasal gland damage caused by the maturing, fourth stage ostertagia larvae. On post-mortem, small nodules 1–2mm in diameter are present on the abomasal mucosal folds, sometimes referred to as a Morocco-leather appearance. Inhibited larvae are visible histologically.

(c) Salmonellosis (often produces dysentery, confirm by culture). Coccidiosis (typically produces tenesmus, passing a mixture of fresh blood, mucus and faeces. Confirm by direct examination for faecal oocysts).

13 (a) A squamous cell carcinoma of the third eyelid (nictitating membrane).

(b) White-faced breeds such as Herefords and others with limited pigmentation around the eye are most commonly affected, due to the association with ultraviolet sunlight. Tumours are also seen on the lower eyelid and corneal-scleral junction.

(c) Using sedation and local anaesthesia, early tumours (such as depicted) can be simply and fully excised. Exteriorise by traction and, using scissors, incise along the residual healthy third eyelid. No suturing is required. A proportion of tumours recur after 1–2 years, although many recover fully. Untreated cases ulcerate, develop secondary infection and may metastasise locally, to the regional lymph nodes or (rarely) the lungs.

14 (a) The urethral opening is sited immediately ventral to the anus, beneath which there is an elongated cleft, exposing a pink mucosa and terminating with the galea glandis, clitoris and a tuft of clitoral hair at the most ventral point. No scrotum is evident.

(b) A pseudohermaphrodite. On rectal examination the initial urethra was thickened, resembling a penis. No uterus or ovaries were palpable. (A true hermaphrodite possesses both ovarian and testicular tissue.)

(c) Freemartinism, caused by placental fusion and interflow of blood between male and female foetuses in early pregnancy.

15 (a) Protrusion of granulation tissue from the medial wall of the left claw.

(b) A longitudinal fissure (vertical sandcrack) with the chronic irritation of secondary infection and/or excess movement leading to the production of granulation tissue.

(c) Amputate the granulation tissue with a hoof-knife, remove under-run hoof from each side of the infected sandcrack and apply a wooden or rubber block to the sound claw, thus resting the affected claw.

16 (a) There is displacement of the mandible between the two central incisors, with haemorrhage at the expanded junction.

(b) Fracture of the mandibular symphysis due to trauma.

(c) Mild cases such as this recover without treatment. If the degree of displacement and motility at the symphysis is more severe, fixation would be required. However, this would only be performed in valuable animals.

17 (a) A bloody exudate lies on the inflamed tracheal mucosa. There is a marked emphysema present, with dilated bullae (A) being particularly apparent beneath the surface of the cardiac lobes. Interlobular septae distended with emphysema (B) are visible in the incised diaphragmatic lobe. There are a few areas of normal (pink) lung remaining, (C) but most of the tissue has an intense deep red pneumonic consolidation.
(b) Respiratory syncytial virus, RSV.
(c) Attention to management, especially reduced stocking density, maintain constant group size and single age group, decrease dust, ammonia and humidity in the atmosphere, and vaccination. Currently the commercially available vaccine is given intramuscularly as two doses 4–6 weeks apart, the first dose being given at three months, to avoid interference with maternally derived colostral immunity. Unfortunately, in a small proportion of herds, vaccination appears to increase the severity of the disease.

18 (a) A red rim of pannus is advancing from the periphery of the cornea. There is a keratitis present, producing corneal opacity. A small black object is embedded in the cornea towards the lateral canthus, surrounded by an area of more intense corneal opacity. Mild lacrimation is evident on the lower lid.
(b) A reaction to a foreign body embedded in the cornea.
(c) Surgical removal of the foreign body under local anaesthesia, using very fine forceps. If this is not successful, in a proportion of cases the foreign body is sloughed naturally (as in this case). In others, the foreign body penetrates into the aqueous, to produce permanent blindness.

19 (a) This is an enlargement of the lateral subcutaneous bursa of the hock, containing a straw-coloured sterile fluid within a synovial membrane.
(b) This is of traumatic origin, most commonly seen in cattle housed in cubicle/free-stall buildings and particularly where there is insufficient bedding or where the floors or divisions are poorly designed, producing many points of impact. It is also commonly seen secondary to lameness, when cows have difficulty in sitting or rising.
(c) If the trauma is removed (e.g. cows turned out to pasture) spontaneous resolution occurs. Continued trauma may result in ulceration of the superficial skin and secondary infection, with a discharging sinus and lameness. This can produce a more severe cellulitis with acute lameness.

20 (a) Actinomycosis ('lumpy jaw'), caused by *Actinomyces bovis*.
(b) Cutaneous actinobacillosis and mandibular abscess. Typically both of these conditions are cutaneous lesions, *viz.*, they move freely within the skin and are not firmly attached to the mandible, whereas actinomycosis produces a rarifying periostitis of the mandible, with secondary soft-tissue reaction. The soft-tissue reaction associated with a chronic actinobacillosis or mandibular abscess may be quite extensive, however, and it may be difficult to distinguish the extent of bone involvement by palpation.
(c) Advanced cases of actinomycosis periostitis produce dysphagia and partial anorexia due to pain on mastication and malalignment of molar teeth. The prognosis for such cases is very poor.

21 (a) Multiple small discrete, raised erythematous foci cover the mucosa. Some are pustular.
(b) Pustular vulvovaginitis, caused by the Infectious Bovine Rhinotracheitis (IBR) virus.

(c) IBR can cause one or more of the following: an acute upper respiratory tract infection, with a necrotising laryngotracheitis; a purulent conjunctivitis; a pustular balanoprosthitis and abortion. Control is by vaccination, annual doses of intranasal vaccine being required.

22 (a) On the lateral curvature of the right claw the white line is irregular and at one point has been impacted with black debris. An area of haemorrhage is present at a similar point on the left claw. The sole horn has a yellow, waxy appearance and is of poor quality. Both heels are lowered, with heel necrosis present, and the toes have been shortened by foot-trimming.
(b) Acidosis, associated with high-concentrate, low-fibre diets, concentrates containing a low level of digestible fibre, and infrequent feeding of concentrates, leading to larger quantities at each feed. Environmental factors include feet continually wet, especially in corrosive slurry, excessive standing on unyielding surfaces and sudden movements, leading to physical tearing of the wall from the sole at the white line.
(c) If left, the impaction could resolve spontaneously, or it might penetrate deeper to produce a white line abscess. Preventive hoof-trimming and removal of the lesion is the best option.

23 (a) A retropharyngeal abscess, confirmed by paracentesis and aspiration of thick, off-white pus.
(b) Either from percutaneous penetration by sharp, infected objects, e.g. thorns or, more commonly, as a result of pharyngeal damage, for example, ingestion of sharp fragments of wood or accidental trauma when using drenching guns, balling guns or a probang.
(c) Lance the abscess at its most dependant part, to produce a large opening and drain the pus. Investigate the depths of the lesion for possible residual foreign bodies. Flush with antiseptic solutions, on alternate days, for a week.

24 (a) Pseudocowpox, caused by paravaccinia virus.
(b) Yes—milker's nodules.
(c) Although the lesion appears raw and rough, it is not particularly painful and does not normally interfere with milking. Spontaneous resolution occurs in 1–2 months, although as immunity is short-lived, repeated attacks may occur every 2–3 years. It is likely that infection is endemic in this herd and that future batches of incoming heifers will also become affected. Infection is spread during milking.

25 (a) Oral necrobacillosis, caused by *Fusobacterium necrophrum* infection and sometimes referred to as diptheria.
(b) i) Dorsum of tongue (calf diptheria), producing pyrexia, salivation and regurgitation of ingested food.
   ii) In the cheek, producing an external nodular swelling of the skin, with ulceration on the buccal surface.
   iii) On the larynx. Affected animals develop dyspnoea, with a pronounced roaring breathing (stridor), but in the early stages remain bright and eat well.
   iv) Ulcers on the rumen mucosa following acidosis.
   v) Hepatic abscessation (often the result of rumen acidosis) leading to depressed performance.
   vi) Interdigital cleft (interdigital necrobacillosis), known colloquially as 'foul' or 'foot rot', producing lameness.

26 (a) A purulent discharging sinus in the ligamentum nuchae.

(b) Continued trauma, e.g. against a badly positioned and/or sharp-edged feed barrier. Initially causing a bursitis at this site, continued trauma of the soft fluctuating swelling leads to its rupture and secondary infection.

(c) Repeated flushing with warm, antiseptic solutions assists recovery. Discharging dorsally, the lesion drains very poorly and construction of an additional ventral drainage point is often beneficial. The initial traumatic factor should be removed. However, lesions are very slow to heal; in this particular cow it took almost a year.

27 (a) The tailhead is raised and the wings of the ileum (the pelvic tuber coxae) are elevated above the level of the dorsal lumbar spine.

(b) Sacroiliac subluxation, leading to rotation of the pelvis on the caudal spine.

(c) Most cases are associated with dystocia, especially foetal oversize and foetal/maternal disproportion. The prognosis can only be fully assessed by rectal palpation. In many cases the sacral spine is depressed ventrally, resulting in a marked reduction of the size of the pelvic canal. Such animals continue to feed and grow normally, but should not be retained for breeding.

28 (a) Middle-ear infection.

(b) Meningitis. However, meningitis cases generally show a more pronounced illness, with pyrexia, anorexia and lethargy and in advanced cases recumbency and extensor spasm.

(c) Prolonged parenteral antibiotic therapy (e.g. daily for 7–10 days) generally effects a full recovery. In a proportion of cases a purulent discharge is seen from the ear canal, as the abscess ruptures.

29 (a) A horizontal sandcrack (horizontal fissure), leading to shelling of the hoof at the toe.

(b) Horizontal sandcracks result from temporary cessation of horn formation and occur following acute fever or toxaemia, e.g. foot-and-mouth disease, metritis or (in this case) mastitis. Hoof grows distally from the coronary band at approximately 5mm per month. Although the upper (dorsal) edge of the sloughing horn is midway (30–50mm) between toe and coronet (average length 70mm) the ventral edge of the new horn will be further from the coronet, probably 40–45mm. The cause of the sandcrack therefore occurred $40 \div 5 = 8$ months ago.

(c) Often none. Many toes will slough without producing significant lameness. If lameness occurs, due to excess movement or secondary infection, remove the loose horn and apply a rubber or wooden block to the sound claw.

30 (a) Corneal opacity, due to pannus extending from the corneoscleral junction to a central perforated corneal ulcer. The corneal ulcer is plugged by the protruding iris to produce a staphyloma.

(b) Infectious bovine keratoconjunctivitis (IBK = New Forest Eye) caused by *Moraxella bovis*.

(c) Exposure to flies, ultraviolet light, warm humid environment, white-faced cattle, high stocking density, and increased animal–animal contact, e.g. at tightly packed feed troughs.

31 (a) Malignant oedema (necrotic cellulitis), an acute, subcutaneous infection caused by a range of clostridial species, especially *Clostridium septicum*.

(b) Cutaneous urticaria (blaine) may produce pyrexia, anorexia and salivation, but the lesions are typically bilateral and often extend also to the neck and remainder of the body. Trauma, producing oedema from bruising, is likely to be non-pyrexic and would leave superficial scarring. Abscess formation and haematomas are generally more localised and non-pyrexic.

(c) Aggressive antibiotic therapy, using daily or twice daily parenteral penicillin or tetracycline at high dosage will effect a cure in mild cases. More advanced cases develop extensive subcutaneous abscessation, often extending down the neck to the brisket and forelimbs. Death may result from toxaemia (as occurred in this cow).

32 (a) There is an open, discharging wound at the point of the tuber coxae, the wing of the pelvic ileum.

(b) Trauma, leading to fracture and sequestration of a small fragment of bone. The trauma is typically due to a fall onto a hard surface, poor cubicle design and/or cows pushing through crowded doorways.

(c) Haematomas may develop at this site. More commonly, ileal wing fractures remain closed, the fragment of bone being pulled downwards by the fascia lata, to produce a typical 'dropped pin-bone' or 'dropped hip'. Such lesions have no clinical significance, apart from their appearance.

33 (a) Digital dermatitis.

(b) It is most probably a bacterial infection, but the cause is unknown. Bacteroides species have been suggested.

(c) Removal of superficial debris and application of an oxytetracycline/gentian-violet aerosol produces effective resolution of the lesion. Control is based on claw hygiene, especially when housed, and the use of tetracycline or dimetridazole footbaths. Formalin is generally found to be of limited value.

34 (a) Gross enlargement of the left upper leg, with a haemorrhagic necrosis of the musculature, sharply contrasting with normal pale muscle on the right leg.

(b) Blackleg, caused by *Clostridium chauvoei*.

(c) *Clostridium chauvoei* is a ubiquitous soil organism and is present in the intestinal tract of many cattle. Disease is thought to occur only when suitable anaerobic conditions are present in the muscle, e.g. deep bruising. Vaccination provides good control. On this farm, cattle had been vaccinated prior to turnout for the previous 15 years. Unfortunately, this particular group was overlooked.

35 (a) A metacarpal mid-shaft chip fracture, producing a sequestrum.

(b) By Xray and/or probe and exploration of the area. In this case the sequestrated fragment was clearly visible on Xray.

(c) Removal of the bone fragment under deep anaesthesia results in a rapid recovery from the lameness. Although easily seen under Xray, the bone chip may, on occasions, be difficult to locate and remove surgically.

36 (a) Irregular deep red pannus formation is progressing circumferentially from the corneoscleral junction. White plaques on the inner surface of the cornea (Descemet's membrane) contribute to the general opacity.

(b) Bovine iritis (also known as uveitis or iridocyclitis).

(c) Bovine iritis has been associated with *Listeria monocytogenes* infection and the feeding of big-bale silage, especially from round feeders.

37 (a) i) Recumbency.

ii) Bulging anus under tail and absence of faeces due to rectal atony.

iii) Mild bloat (ruminal atony).

iv) Characteristic 'S-bend' posture of the neck, thought to be a self-righting response as the animal attempts to avoid full lateral recumbency.

(b) i) High dietary calcium prepartum.

ii) Low dietary calcium and vitamin D immediately post-partum.

iii) Older cows.

iv) High yields.

v) Excessive prepartum feeding, leading to overfat cows, partial liver insufficiency and increased yields immediately post-partum.

vi) Excessively high or low dietary magnesium intakes prepartum.

vii) High pasture intakes prepartum.

(c) Solutions of 40% calcium borogluconate are best not given subcutaneously, as they are irritant and may produce a sterile abscess at the site of injection.

38 (a) The right claw is grossly swollen above the coronet, with hyperaemia of the underlying skin. Early separation of the coronary band from the skin is visible at the heel-horn junction. A sole ulcer at the typical site of the same claw has a red, raw and granulating central area, producing a purulent discharge over the soiled solar horn. A wooden block has been fixed to the left claw.

(b) An initial sole ulcer which has led to infection of the deep pedal tissues, for example the navicular bursa, or navicular bone or, most likely, from the degree of swelling, infection of the corono-pedal (third phalangeal) joint.

(c) A variety of treatments is available, producing either removal or drainage of the infected focus. These include:

i) Digit amputation.

ii) Deep pedal curettage, in which a 2–3cm diameter opening is incised through the solar horn and laminae, removing all necrotic material (including the navicular bone if infected).

iii) Drill from the lateral coronary band medially into the interdigital space, insert a perforated plastic tube and regularly flush the infected joint.

Provided that cases are treated early, before advanced ascending swelling and infection occurs, and provided that extensive antibiotic therapy is given, the prognosis is reasonable for most cases. Using methods (ii) and (iii), the coronopedal joint eventually becomes ankylosed, leading to permanent rotation of the claw and elevation of the toe. This will probably necessitate periodic corrective foot trimming.

39 (a) Listeriosis, a bacterial meningoencephalitis caused by *Listeria monocytogenes*.

(b) Other forms of meniningitis or meningoencephalitis, for example Aujeszky's, non-specific bacterial infections and abscesses; lead poisoning; botulism; BSE; hypo-magnesaemia.

(c) Abortion; mastitis; iritis. Listeria is ubiquitous, being carried by most domestic birds, animals and wildlife.

40 (a) Although approximately normal in size, with no sharp demarcation between scrotal and inguinal tissue, the skin of the scrotum shows a superficial slough of dry, necrotic areas, with healthy new skin beneath.

(b) Faulty application of the Burdizzo bloodless castrator. If the two crush marks form a continuous line across the scrotal neck, skin necrosis results.

41 (a) Cut the toes back to equal length and approximately 70mm from toe to coronet.

(b) Remove solar hoof from the toe, so that the white line reappears and the hoof is tilted forward, to give a 45° angle between the anterior hoof wall and the floor surface.

(c) Remove the medial ledge of horn (A), ensuring that weight is then taken only by the heels and the hoof wall, extending laterally from the heel to the toe and a short distance caudally on the medial wall.

(d) Pay particular attention to the lateral left claw, so that its size no longer exceeds that of the medial claw.

42 (a) Prolapse (proptosis) of the eyeball, which protrudes well beyond the lids. There is intense congestion and oedema of the sclera.

(b) Trauma to the head.

(c) Repulsion of the eyeball under general anaesthesia, followed by surgical closure of the lids for a further 7 days, resulted in full recovery.

43 (a) A bruised udder, of traumatic origin.

(b) Gangrenous mastitis. Milk from both quarters should be carefully drawn to check. Affected animals generally show severe systemic illness, however.

(c) For the majority of cases, no treatment is required and the condition resolves spontaneously over 4–6 weeks. If excessive oedema produces discomfort or makes milking difficult, diuretics can prove beneficial.

44 (a) Lumbar spondylosis. Osteophyte formation along the ventral surface of the lumbar vertebrae leads to intense pain and restricted movement. The hind limbs are placed well back and the lumbar spine dipped, in an attempt to relieve the pain.

(b) The prognosis is hopeless. The condition progressively deteriorates until the cow becomes recumbent and may be considered as part of the 'downer cow' syndrome.

45 (a) A fibropapilloma.

(b) Penile fibropapillomata are thought to be of viral origin. They are most commonly seen in younger bulls and especially in those closely confined in groups.

(c) A significant proportion of mild cases slowly resolve without treatment and many are probably never detected. More advanced cases lead to penile prolapse and/or post-coital bleeding and require removal. If pedunculated, simple ligation is adequate, otherwise surgical removal is required. The prognosis is generally good and the vast majority of bulls can return to use in natural service.

46 (a) Bovine spongiform encephalopathy.

(b) Grinding teeth, excessive licking of the nostrils, a shivering spasmodic contraction of the skin muscles, progressive ataxia, change in behaviour, apprehension, e.g. fear of walking through narrow doorways and occasionally unprovoked violent behaviour, e.g. kicking wildly at the milking machine.

(c) Spongiform encephalopathies (originally called slow virus infections, but 'virus' is a misnomer). Other diseases in this group include scrapie in sheep, kuru and Creutzfeldt-Jakob in man; transmissible mink encephalopathy; chronic wasting disease of kudu and eland and feline spongiform encephalopathy.

47 (a) Bilateral obturator paralysis. The degree of limb abduction is so severe that it is most probable that either both femurs have fractured or both hips have dislocated.

(b) Dystocia, especially when associated with foetal oversize or foetal-maternal disproportion is a common cause of obturator paralysis. A similar syndrome can occur when a cow 'does the splits' following introduction onto slippery concrete, or when a heifer is bullied and knocked following introduction into a dairy herd.

(c) In this case, hopeless. Less severe cases of partial obturator paralysis should be hobbled and maintained on deep straw or some other form of non-slip flooring to prevent complications.

48 (a) Prolapse of the uterus, cervix and vagina.

(b) Most cases of uterine prolapse occur within a few hours of calving and are typically seen in older cows, following the delivery of large calves or dystocia, and may be associated with hypocalcaemia.

(c) Following repulsion and correction, the prognosis for uterine prolapse is good, although there is a slightly increased chance of the condition recurring at the next parturition. Although it is relatively easy to repel a combined prolapse of uterus, cervix and vagina, the prognosis is poor as a significant proportion of cases (this cow included) die within 24 hours from internal haemorrhage, following rupture of a major blood vessel.

49 (a) A teat cistern granuloma or 'pea'. Irregular rubbery masses of fibrocollagenous material ('peas') may pass down the teat sinus with the flow of milk and then obstruct the sphincter.

(b) Smaller granulomata can be manually expressed under pressure. Others require local anaesthesia of the teat end (most easily obtained by infusing 20–30ml local anaesthetic directly into the teat cistern) and either dilation with a McCleans knife, or removal of the granuloma by means of crocodile forceps or a teat spiral.

(c) The prognosis for free-floating granulomata is excellent. However, a proportion are attached to the inner teat cistern wall by a membrane and these are very difficult to remove. Occasionally the membrane itself occludes the sphincter by floating across the sinus orifice. The prognosis is then hopeless.

50 (a) Characteristic 'ten to four' appearance, showing dilation of the dorsal abdomen on the left and the ventral abdomen on the right.

(b) Forestomach obstruction, e.g. typically vagus indigestion and occasionally abomasal and/or omasal torsion.

(c) Hopeless. Best to cull.

51 (a) The lateral vaginal, a branch of the internal pudendal, located bilaterally at the 4 o'clock and 8 o'clock positions, approximately wrist depth into the vagina.

(b) Clamp the bleeding point with artery forceps and suture the forceps into position for 4–5 days. Occasionally both ends of the blood vessel need ligating.

(c) Overfat heifers; oversized foetus; excessively rapid traction allowing insufficient time for vaginal dilation; inadequate lubrication.

52 (a) Bilateral vertical sandcracks, with a broken toe on the right claw.

(b) Dry sandy conditions underfoot lead to loss of the periople, the thin waxy layer which normally covers the hoof. Damage to the coronary band may lead to the production of a localised horn defect.

(c) Simple uninfected sandcracks in cattle often require no treatment. They do not cause lameness and may resolve spontaneously. Infected sandcracks produce acute lameness. The fissure must be opened with a hoof-knife, to achieve drainage of pus, and the affected claw is best rested by applying a wooden or rubber block to the sole of the sound claw.

53 (a) Spina bifida and arthrogryposis of the tail.
(b) Absence of the dorsal portion of the spinal column allows protrusion of the cord and meninges (a myelomeningocoele).

54 (a) Intestinal aplasia, a congenital defect in which a portion of the intestine is absent. Intestinal contents pass directly into the abdomen, leading to peritonitis.
(b) Segmental asplasia. Jejunum, ileum, colon, rectum or anus may be involved, leading to intestinal obstruction and progressive abdominal distension. The clinical syndrome is slower in onset than intestinal aplasia, particularly if the lower gut is affected, and the calf may suckle normally for the first 2–4 days of life before any obvious discomfort is evident.

55 (a) A mammary (milk) vein abscess.
(b) Use of the vein for intravenous administration of calcium borogluconate in the treatment of hypocalcaemia.
(c) Erosion into the mammary vein can produce fatal haemorrhage. Pyaemia arising from the abscess can lead to valvular endocarditis.

56 (a) 'Dropped udder', caused by rupture of the median suspensory ligament, usually at the point of its attachment to the abdominal wall.
(b) Hereditary, and prepartum overfeeding leading to excessive udder engorgement and oedema.

57 (a) Psoroptic mange, caused by *Psoroptes ovis*. Mites were demonstrated on microscopic examination of skin scrapings. Sarcoptic mange is similar in appearance.
(b) Ivermectin injection and pour-on organophosphorus preparations (e.g. 20% phosmet) could both be used. Organophosphorus treatment would need to be repeated after 2 weeks to kill newly hatched mites, as it is not effective against eggs. Because of the persistency of ivermectin, repeat treatments are much less important.

58 (a) A variety of names have been used, including udder seborrhoea, necrotic dermatitis and intertrigo.
(b) Most probably an ischaemic necrosis of the skin caused by peripartum mammary oedema. The condition most commonly develops soon after parturition.
(c) As it is an ischaemic necrosis, remove necrotic tissue (debraidement) by washing with warm antiseptic solutions and apply antiseptic ointment or glycerine.

59 (a) Excessive hind limb abduction ('splaylegging' or 'doing the splits') in a freshly calved cow, due to partial obturator nerve paralysis and/or by walking on slippery concrete flooring. Bullying by other cows on entry into the milking herd is also important.
(b) Apply hobbles to prevent further splaying. Move advanced cases onto a straw-based surface.

60 (a) Bilateral exophthalmos and convergent strabismus.

(b) Strabismus with exophthalmos is a congenital inherited condition, although most cases do not become apparent until the animal is at least 3 months old and often not until 6–9 months.

(c) Guarded. The condition progresses with age and vision becomes impaired.

61 (a) Congenital bilateral contracted tendons and knee (carpal) flexion.

(b) A proportion of cases are inherited through an autosomal recessive gene. Others are thought to be due to abnormal *in utero* foetal posture, often associated with foetal oversize.

(c) The majority of cases of congenital *fetlock* flexion recover spontaneously. Knee flexion (as in this case) is slower to resolve and may need supportive splinting, sometimes combined with flexor tendonectomy. A proportion of advanced cases do not recover.

62 (a) An umbilical granuloma.

(b) If left untreated, the granuloma may persist as an irritating lesion and a possible source of pyaemia for weeks, or even months. Simple ligation, with parenteral antibiotic cover, repeated at weekly intervals until the lesion sloughs, is effective treatment.

63 (a) In this calf a chronic navel infection had eroded through the ventral rumen wall, leading to leakage of rumen contents. Differential diagnoses include spontaneous rupture of a navel abscess and a recto-urethral fistula. The latter condition is likely to be seen within the first few days of life and faecal soiling would be evident around the prepuce and not cranial to it.

(b) Navel abscesses are easily flushed and drained and recover well with parenteral antibiotic cover. Calves with recto-urethral fistulae should be culled. Surgical closure of rumenal fistulae is not easy, due to seepage of rumenal fluid impeding healing and should only be attempted in valuable animals.

64 (a) Rotavirus, coronavirus and/or cryptosporidia.

(b) Surveys have shown that approximately 80% of all primary infectious causes of calf scour are of viral origin. Bacterial infections tend to cause either acute disease (e.g. *E. coli* or *Cl. welchii*) in younger calves, or a higher mortality in older calves (e.g. salmonellosis).

(c) Coronavirus and rotavirus are ubiquitous infections, that is they are found on the majority of farms and as such most calves are exposed to infection, establishing an immunity within the first 1–3 weeks of life. Only a proportion develop disease (i.e. scouring). Control is based on:

   i) reducing the challenge dose of infection, e.g. all-in:all-out housing systems, avoid high stocking densities, maintain ample bedding and general hygiene in housing and feeding.

   ii) continuing to feed colostrum at a low level for the first 2–3 weeks of life. Even in unvaccinated animals there is likely to be sufficient colostral immunoglobulin to afford some surface intestinal protection. A commercial rotavirus/K99 *E.coli* vaccine, administered to the dam prepartum, provides additional immunoglobulin protection.

   iii) minimising environmental and nutritional stresses which could exacerbate the disease.

65 (a) Two perforated ulcers, circumscribed by off-white diptheritic material are seen on the inflamed mucosal surface of a dilated abomasum.

(b) A large proportion of veal calves are found to have asymptomatic ulcers at slaughter. Abomasal dilation is commonly seen clinically, but ulcer perforation is relatively rare.

(c) Hunger and long periods between feeds, leading to excess abomasal acidity, plus ingestion of forage which, in the pre-ruminant calf, passes undigested into the abomasum, are the main suggested causes. Abomasal dilation is associated with a rise in pH and a bacterial proliferation in abomasal fluid.

66 (a) Pronounced tenesmus, with an open anal sphincter and exposed rectal mucosa, allowing the passage of small quantities of blood and mucus only. Black faecal staining from the thighs and perineum down to the hocks. Hair loss on the medial aspect of the legs, indicating more prolonged faecal soiling.

(b) Coccidiosis, caused by *Eimeria zuernii* or *E. bovis*.

(c) Disease is associated with faecal-oral contamination and hence occurs most commonly in crowded, unhygienic conditions. Adult suckler cows may be carriers. Oral treatment with amprolium or sulphonamides is usually effective, but some advanced cases are fatal.

67 (a) Rumenitis, leading to poor rumen function and inefficient digestion.

(b) Oesophageal groove closure defects and unsuitable solid food offered to the preruminant calf, e.g. high-starch cereal rations causing acidosis. Incomplete oesophageal groove closure is primarily a management problem, for example, associated with incorrect bucket or teat height, irregular feeding times, variable temperatures of the milk feed, stress during feeding, etc.

(c) Removal of solid feed followed by intense oral and parenteral antibiotic therapy, combined with 4 days of oral electrolytes and then a liquid diet only for 2 weeks, prior to slow reintroduction of solid food, sometimes assists resolution. However, many cases recur and require the construction of a permanent rumenal fistula. Fistulated calves generally respond and improve quite rapidly.

68 (a) Bilateral necrosis of the ear tips, with loss of more than half the pinna.

(b) Ergot poisoning; post-septicaemic necrosis, e.g. following an *E. coli* or, as in the calf, *Salmonella dublin* infection; a multifocal progressive bilateral necrosis caused by *Actinomyces pyogenes* can occur, but this typically affects the whole pinna and not just the tip.

(c) At this stage, very little. The source of the ergot should be investigated and, if identified, removed: septicaemia would have occurred some 4–6 weeks previously and no further treatment is required. Localised *A. pyogenes* infections require topical lavage and antiseptic therapy.

69 (a) Extensive hair-loss around the muzzle and lower jaw, partial hair-loss around the eye with thick, light brown discharge matted into the surrounding hair, and salivation.

(b) Alopecia of this nature is occasionally seen in calves fed milk substitute and results from fat globules adhering to the skin over the muzzle. The causes include inadequate mixing of the milk substitute, feeding at too low a temperature (preventing full dispersion of fat), calves which drink very slowly, and possibly low-grade rumenitis.

70 (a) Large areas of dry, hard necrotic white skin are sloughing, to reveal a new epidermis, with areas of granulation tissue beneath. This heifer is affected by photosensitisation (photosensitive dermatitis).

(b) Photoreactive chemicals accumulating under the skin convert ultraviolet light into thermal energy, leading to inflammatory changes which cause initial pyrexia, generalised discomfort and an oedematous thickening of the white skin, then later an ischaemic necrosis and cutaneous slough. Only white areas are affected, since black skin prevents the absorption of sunlight. In cattle, the principle photoreactive agents are porphyrins and phylloerythrins, the latter being a normal breakdown product of chlorophyll that is not metabolised further. These result from liver damage arising from the ingestion of a wide range of plants and chemicals, e.g., St. Johns Wort, Lantana and the fungus *Pithomyces chartarum*.

(c) At this advanced stage of the condition it is doubtful if any treatment is worthwhile, apart from housing by day to prevent further exposure to ultraviolet light. Anti-inflammatories and antihistamines are useful in the early stages.

71 (a) Chorioptic mange, caused by *Chorioptes bovis*.
(b) Psoroptic, sarcoptic and demodectic mange are all seen.
(c) Treatment is identical to that used for psoroptic mange, see question 57.

72 (a) Lice eggs.
(b) Sucking lice (*Haemotopinus eurysternus, Linognathus vituli* and – in North America – *Solenoptes capillatus*) and biting lice (*Bovicola bovis*).
(c) Biting lice produce pruritis, sucking lice additional anaemia, weightloss and occasionally very heavy infestations can be fatal. Adult lice can be seen with the naked eye as small, beige-coloured, elongated, motile bodies on the skin surface. Clinically infestations are manifest by rubbing, biting or scratching. The hair on the neck of affected calves often develops into vertical lines and, in advanced cases, the skin becomes thickened. Localised areas of alopecia appear as a result of continual biting, licking or scratching.

73 (a) Ringworm.
(b) *Trichophyton verrucosum* is the most common cause in cattle, with *Microsporum* species being occasionally involved. Ringworm is a fungal infection of the superficial keratinised tissues of the hair and skin, producing a dry, scaly dermatitis, with fracture of the hair shafts at epidermal level, leading to localised alopecia.
(c) Lesions are irritant and affected animals rub against posts and feed troughs, where they deposit spores which can remain infective for up to 4 years. Griseofulvin, a fungistat, can be given orally, daily for 7 days, or nystatin, a fungicide, applied as a topical spray.

74 (a) Warble fly, caused by *Hypoderma bovis* and *H. lineatum*.
(b) Warble larvae appear as nodules under the skin from February onwards, emerging to pupate until the end of May.
(c) Air-holes made by feeding larvae render this area of the hide, normally the most valuable, useless for leather; large numbers of larvae feeding leads to discomfort, depressed production, weightloss and a degree of pyrexia in heavy infestations. The noise of the adult fly approaching to lay its eggs, during May–August, often induces fear or even panic in cattle, leading to restlessness, reduced grazing and sometimes injury, for example, they damage their teats on wire fences. Finally, occasional larvae die when migrating through the spine (*H. bovis* only), leading to posterior ataxia or paralysis.

75 (a) A haematoma. An abscess, the main differential, would develop more slowly and be a harder and possibly a slightly hot, inflamed and painful structure.
(b) Haematomas are the result of subcutaneous bleeding, caused by trauma and often appear in the areas where skin directly covers bone, e.g. over the pelvis, shoulder and lateral chest.
(c) None. In the majority of cases haematomas resolve spontaneously over 3–6 weeks, leaving only thickened skin folds to indicate their original position. Occasional cases become secondarily infected, due to skin erosion or iatrogenic interference, develop into abscesses and have to be lanced, drained, flushed and given secondary parenteral antibiotic cover.

76 (a) Brachygnathia, or parrot mouth.
(b) Chondrodysplasia (= abnormal growth of cartilage).
(c) Brachygnathia and other jaw abnormalities resulting in defective dental apposition are genetically determined by a recessive gene. Total dwarfism, for example, in Herefords, is a more extreme form of inherited chrondrodysplasia.

ANSWERS

Pigs

77 You suggest that sows which have had more than 7 litters be culled so that total numbers born can be improved and that numbers born dead can be reduced. You suggest a policy of routine culling after litter 7 and, if farrowings are not attended, suggest that also.

78 (a) The problem in this case was due to parvovirus infection, but other causes of foetal death, mummification and stillbirth include enterovirus infections 'SMEDI', leptospirosis, Aujeszky's disease in countries where it occurs and, more recently, in Europe, Porcine Respiratory and Reproductive Syndrome (PRRS) and 'SIRS' (Swine Infertility and Respiratory Syndrome) in North America. In these recent syndromes, piglets are more commonly premature and stillborn.
(b) The diagnosis can be confirmed by the laboratory examination of pleural fluid from stillborn piglets for antibody to parvovirus and the tissues of the mummies for virus.
(c) Confirmation of the diagnosis should be followed by serological testing of the herd for parvovirus antibody. If antibody negative pigs are identified at all, then vaccination should be considered.

79 (a) The disease was pleuropneumonia and the clinical signs are typical of untreated disease. Other pneumonias rarely cause death in this age group. Glassers Disease and Pasteurellosis can both cause mortality, but Bordetellosis, Enzootic Pneumonia and Influenza rarely do so.
(b) Post-mortem examination of the dead animals would confirm the presence of pleuropneumonia with its characteristic lesions of pleurisy and infarction of the lung.

80 The animal has hydronephrosis. It is rather young for polycystic kidneys and in that case would not have the dilated ureters shown here. Urine could pass into the bladder in this case.

81 (a) The faeces is white because villous atrophy has occurred and the piglet is unable to digest and absorb all the milk fat.
(b) Diseases which cause villous atrophy include rotavirus, porcine epidemic diarrhoea, transmissible gastroenteritis (TGE), which caused this problem, and coccidiosis.

82 The sow has mastitis which normally results from ascending infection with *E. coli* or other bacteria:
(a) The sow could be managed by treatment with intravenous oxytocin and intramuscular injection with oxytetracycline or ampicillin daily for 2–3 days.
(b) The piglets could be given access to water or to fluid replacer and, if the sow remained unable to feed them, be given milk replacer by stomach tube or by free access in a dish.

83 (a) The feature concerned is a retained abdominal testicle: it cannot be removed by normal castration if this is practised and may give rise to boar taint in pigs slaughtered at higher weights.
(b) It would render the boar unsuitable for breeding or sale for breeding.

84 The condition shown is a healed fracture of 3 ribs. This is probably incidental but if several pigs were found to be affected, it would be worth enquiring about the circumstances, because there might be welfare implications.

85 The feed has been contaminated by fodder mites which have multiplied in numbers sufficient to render the feed unpalatable. The mites are the pinkish uniform material in the centre of the photograph and can be seen as slowly moving particles when examined closely.

86 (a) The gilt died from *Eubacterium (Corynebacterium) suis* infection. The organism was demonstrated in Gram-stained smears of the urine and by anaerobic culture on horseblood agar after 4 days' anaerobic incubation.
(b) Prevention in the short term would involve intramuscular injection of recently served gilts and sows with penicillin and the routine use in future of antimicrobial washing of the preputial sac of the boar(s) with antimicrobials such as tetracyclines.

87 The pig has died from a twisted bowel. The twist involves both small and large intestine which are intensely congested. The stomach is unaffected.

88 The condition is rectal stricture which accounts for the distended abdomen seen in *Figure 89*. The cause is not always identifiable, but the most consistent one is previous infection with salmonella. The necrotic surface of the ileum shown in *Figure 90* did not involve the proliferation seen in proliferative enteropathy and *S. typhimurium* phage type 204c was isolated from it.

89 The cause might have been Vitamin E deficiency or Mulberry Heart disease. The histological findings suggested Vitamin E deficiency.

90 Yes, in this case there is firm evidence for a crushing injury, as there is a large blood clot in the torn mesentery from ante-mortem injury and bruising of the abdominal wall (not shown).

91 (a) The cause of death was bleeding from a gastric ulcer in the pars oesophagea of the stomach.
(b) The pig might have survived if identified as affected in life, separated from its fellows and given fluids and anti-ulcer drugs.

92 (a) The pigs have 'colitis'. There is no evidence for the presence of small intestinal causes of mild diarrhoea such as Proliferative Enteropathy or of swine dysentery, spirochaetal diarrhoea or parasitic infections in the colon. The apparently normal-looking colonic mucosa and contents are typical of the findings in this condition. Even histological lesions may be absent in many cases. No pathogens can be demonstrated in the contents. The presence of cryptosporidia, rotavirus, TGE, PED, salmonella, entero-toxigenic *Clostridium perfringens* type A and *Yersinia enterocolitica* should be eliminated.
(b) Treatment with tiamulin, dimetridazole or lincomycin may be successful. The inclusion of growth permitters such as avoparcin or the use of zinc oxide at 2,000 ppm may be effective. Changes in the feed and the use of meal rather than pellets may be of value.

93 (a) The castration has been carried out carelessly. There is infection of the castration wounds (top) and backbleeding and infection in the abdomen.
(b) Training of the stockman should take place or the unit should be encouraged to abandon castration, if the eventual purchaser of the pigs will still buy them.

94 The piglet in *Figure 98*. Its lungs are plum coloured and sink in water.

95 The condition is 'humpy-back' or kyphosis and on this farm was present to a slight extent in some of the breeding stock. It was most prominent in pigs kept in kennelled pens with a tiny entry hole. There was also histological and serological evidence of Talfan Disease. The conditions noted above might all have contributed to the kyphosis seen.

96 (a) The pigs have sarcoptic mange.
(b) The easiest way to confirm the presence of the disease is to take scrapings from the inner surface of the pig's ear and examine them and any wax crusts recovered under a warm lamp. Mites will be seen scurrying about when viewed with a hand lens. Alternatively, the waxy material can be cleared with 40% potassium hydroxide for 10 minutes and then viewed with the low-power lens of a microscope, when the mites will be obvious.

97 (a) The problem is louse (*Haematopinus suis*) infestation.
(b) The presence of lice can be confirmed by finding the large blackish adults on the skin, particularly in the ears and on the extremities. Feeding lesions may be present in the ears and eggs are present on the hairs inside the ears and on the neck, just behind the ears, in longstanding infestations. Treatment may be carried out with ivermectin, diazinon, coumaphos, phosmet, deltamethrin or amitraz applied in the appropriate manner.

98 (a) The piglet is suffering from vulval necrosis. This may be caused by damage to the vulva by poor quality flooring, especially expanded metal which can shred the vulva. Hyperoestrogenism of maternal or mycotoxic origin may predispose by causing vulval hypertrophy.
(b) The consequences are rarely significant for slaughter pigs, but there may be scarring or the formation of adhesions which reduce the animals' value for breeding.

99 (a) The problem is due to poor sow condition.
(b) It can be corrected by ensuring that the gilts are fed adequately and are in good condition (condition score 2–3) at farrowing and that they receive adequate feed during lactation. If they cannot eat enough to maintain body condition, consider the use of a high-energy ration. Continue this for at least the first week after weaning. Ensure that gilts and dry sows are in accommodation kept at the appropriate temperature (20°C) and that there are no draughts. It may also be of value to weigh sows and to ensure that they gain at least 12.5kg and remain in good condition. Outdoor sows may require worming.

100 Acute *Ascaris suum* infection. The animals have been infected with very large numbers of eggs from the uncleaned pen and were in the migration phase at the time the photographs were taken. The lungs and liver show evidence of tracks made by the larvae.

101 Lameness was caused by epiphyseolysis which results from poor ossification of the femoral head due to osteochondrosis dissecans. The actual avulsion of the femoral head results from awkward movements resulting from riding in gilts approaching sexual maturity, bad flooring or transport.

102 The porcine stress syndrome. Heavily muscled pigs often carry the stress gene and this may cause death in hot conditions (in excess of 28°C). Altered muscles may be seen in the ham, the longissimus dorsi and the shoulders.

103 (a) The disease is exudative epidermitis (greasy pig disease) caused by *Staphylococcus hyicus*. The lesions shown in *Figure 113* are typical as are the post mortem changes. The renal lesions result from dehydration.
(b) The condition can be treated by penicillin, ampicillin or lincomycin injection coupled with washing with a disinfectant such as chlorhexidine or hexocil. Early treatment in the farrowing house prevents the disease entering the flat deck and the removal of any projecting metal and correction of temperature and humidity reduce the chance of its occurrence.

104 The cause is Ascaris impaction of the bile duct. This occasionally occurs in heavily infected pigs.

105 (a) The cause was overgrowth of the sole.
(b) It could have been trimmed, the sow put through a footbath and then she could have been kept on firmer, more abrasive flooring.

106 (a) The disease is proliferative enteropathy (PE) and the animal has died from the haemorrhagic form of the disease.
(b) It may be treated by medication with oxytetracycline or chlortetracycline for 1–2 weeks followed by an interval of 3 weeks and then another course of treatment. Other antimicrobials, such as neomycin and trimethoprim sulphonamide, may also be used.

107 The disease is swine dysentery. It is unaffected by tetracycline treatment, and typical mucoid stools can be seen when the animals do not defaecate on slats.

108 (a) The condition is pityriasis rosea and it is not life-threatening.
(b) It is unsightly but should disappear by the time of slaughter and is associated with slightly slower growth at the worst.

109 The cause of death was a strangulated inguinal hernia. There had been Glasser's Disease in the group and this animal had developed adhesions with fatal consequences.

110 The animal is too thin, possibly because she is being kept in a group and is not getting enough food and possibly because of the uncorrected weight loss from this or previous litters. She is suffering from the thin-sow syndrome and this will have reproductive consequences (*see* Question **99**).

111 Gangrenous metritis. The carcase was already decomposing and *C. perfringens* type A was isolated in pure and profuse culture from the uterine lumen and from the decomposing piglets it contained.

112 The underlying cause of this 'colitis' problem is proliferative enteropathy restricted to the large intestine. The 'colitis' should be treated as a case of PE (*see* Question **106**).

113 Thirst. They have insufficient water for their requirements and at least one had crystalluria as a result. Instructions were given to replace the ring with a drinker of sufficient capacity.

114 (a) The condition is a form of contact dermatitis which occurs when chronically dysenteric animals in dirty conditions are treated with tiamulin, lincomycin or, sometimes, with tylosin. Some may die.
(b) All affected animals recover if medication is discontinued and the animals are washed with water. The pen must also be cleaned out. Lesions take several days to fade.

115 The cause was a strangulated umbilical hernia in which the small intestine had become trapped.

116 The tail has been caught in the expanded metal of the pen floor and has been damaged.

117 A wallow fed by a water spray. This allows animals to cool down and thus prevents mortality from heat stress and encourages appetite.

118 (a) The lesion is caused by a rough back-plate to the stall which may also be too short.
(b) The owner should be advised to remove all old (and therefore larger) sows from such crates and to check for rough edges. In the long term, back-plates which are curved to allow for greater body-length may be installed.

119 Nothing. In spite of their misery, they will soon recover. They have just been tatooed with their ear numbers.

120 They are visiting a High Health Herd and are dressed in the farm's own clothing and boots in order to reduce the risk of transmission of disease. They will also have refrained from visiting other pigs for a period specified by the herd's veterinarian, usually 48 hours but sometimes longer.

121 (a) You suspect a vesicular disease such as Foot-and-Mouth Disease or Swine Vesicular Disease.
(b) You do not leave the farm but notify the local Ministry of Agriculture Veterinarian and await his arrival. Until he arrives you do not allow anyone else to leave the unit. The disease shown here was Foot-and-Mouth Disease. It may affect other species on the farm and causes mortality in sucking piglets, both features of this disease not found in Swine Vesicular Disease.

122 By treating all pigs on both sides of the partition. Infection will be spread by the drainage or by cleaning to all animals. Treatment of the single affected pens alone will lead to the development of disease elsewhere within a few days. Severely affected pigs may be treated parenterally with tiamulin or lincomycin or given dimetridazole, tiamulin or lincomycin in the drinking water. The remainder of the animals may be treated at therapeutic level in the feed. This treatment should be accompanied by cleaning, hosing down of the dunging channel and disinfection of the dunging channel and any contaminated areas inside the pens, especially water bowls. The pigs concerned should not be sent for slaughter until the withdrawal period is complete. Restocking should be carried out one side at a time after thorough cleaning. The scraper should be thoroughly disinfected before use in another house or a separate implement used.

123 The central black area is blood clot. The animal died suddenly having developed haemopericardium as a result of aortic rupture.

124 Tuberculosis. This is usually avian and can be confirmed by Ziehl-Neelsen-stained smears in which acid-fast bacteria can be seen, and by culture. As *Mycobacterium avium* and the mammalian tubercle bacilli are potential human pathogens, this examination should be carried out under appropriate safety conditions.

125 Congenital meningoencephalocoele. It is usually lethal.

126 (a) The disease is thrombocytopaenic purpura but the lesions resemble closely those of classical or African swine fever. The history and the absence of fevered pigs are typical of thrombocytopaenic purpura and make those diseases unlikely, but in view of the importance of these conditions the Ministry of Agriculture should be notified and you should not leave the farm until the state veterinarian arrives.
(b) For thrombocytopaenic purpura, Vitamin K injection may improve the remaining affected pigs. The old sow should be culled, or, if she has to be reused, she should be bred to a different boar. If this is not possible, the piglets should not receive colostrum from her but should receive a colostral supplement and be placed on another sow until all colostrum has been consumed by that sow's litter.

127 (a) The disease is classical swine fever (hog cholera).
(b) The disease should be reported to the Ministry of Agriculture and no-one should leave the farm until after a state veterinarian arrives. Carcases will be removed to a Veterinary Investigation Centre for further examination or samples will be taken on the farm. Thorough disinfection will be necessary before anyone can leave the unit. Samples for further investigation should include spleen, kidney, clotted and unclotted blood, pancreas, and lymph nodes. In view of the difficulty of distinguishing between this disease and African swine fever, duplicate samples will be sent for examination for both diseases. The pigs will be slaughtered if the disease is confirmed.

128 (a) This is a case of vegetative endocarditis.
(b) Organisms commonly present in the lesions include *Erysipelothrix rhusiopathiae* for which vaccination should be introduced, streptococci, staphylococci and, occasionally, organisms such as *Actinobacillus suis*.

129 The condition is ringworm.

130 (a) The findings are suggestive of electrocution as pathological fractures from nutritional causes should not affect animals suddenly and in such numbers.
(b) You should check electrical wiring with care and especially anything which may be connected to pen furniture such as drinkers and railings. Such fittings may be live.

131 (a) The piglet is in a position typical of splayleg and will eventually recover if able to suck.
(b) The survival of affected animals is enhanced if the hind legs are kept together with a rubber band or tape and if they are given supplementary feeding for the first few days of life.

132 (a) The pigs have progressive atrophic rhinitis.
(b) The bony changes are unlikely to resolve entirely, but treatment of the group may eliminate residual populations of the toxigenic *Pasteurella multocida* type D and any

associated pneumonia. Vaccination at this stage cannot be justified. Further pigs should not be purchased from this supplier unless he controls the condition by vaccination or treatment as the growth rate of affected pigs may remain lower than would be expected.

133 (a) The animal has died from pneumonic pasteurellosis. There is no pleurisy and no necrotic lesions of the type expected in pleuropneumonia. A profuse culture of *P. multocida* type A was isolated and *A. pleuropneumoniae* had never been isolated from the herd.

(b) Treatment with parenteral penicillin, ampicillin or oxytetracycline could be used in individuals and the group treated with feed or the water medicated with chlortetracycline or oxytetracycline. In theory it is possible to vaccinate pigs at risk but most pasteurella vaccines currently contain type D antigens and few if any contain type A. Improving the ventilation, all in all out housing and feed medication of groups of pigs entering the accommodation may all help.

134 (a) The animal had salt poisoning through being unable to reach water during its illness combined with the dehydrating effects of severe pleuropneumonia.

(b) The gradual recovery suggests salt poisoning as does the central blindness. Histological evidence of an eosinophilic meningitis was found at post-mortem examination and confirms the identity of the disease.

135 (a) The piglet has joint ill, a septic arthritis.

(b) This is usually caused by *Streptococcus suis* type 1, but may occasionally be caused by staphylococci, *Haemophilus parasuis* or *Actinobacillus suis*.

136 (a) The history and clinical signs are typical of pantothenic acid deficiency.

(b) The ataxic animals will probably not recover and should be slaughtered. The goosestepping animals will recover and can be treated with Vitamin B complexes in the first instance. The disease can be prevented by including calcium pantothenate in the ration at the rate of 10–12g/tonne after the mix has cooled.

137 (a) The disease is pig pox.

(b) There is no treatment. It occurs sporadically in herds and is suppressed by maternal immunity. The spread of infection can be reduced in an affected herd by thorough disinfection and all-in all-out husbandry, and by reducing sharp or abrasive surfaces in accommodation such as flat decks.

138 (a) The condition is oral necrobacillosis.

(b) *Fusobacterium necrophorum* and other fusobacteria colonise the lesions caused by careless tooth clipping. When extensive, these infections lead to death, as in this case.

139 (a) The disease is Aujeszky's Disease and the death of other species is commonplace. If this did not occur, the Porcine Respiratory and Reproductive Syndrome (PRRS) should be considered, although the nervous signs are unlikely in that disease.

(b) In Great Britain the disease has been eradicated and a breakdown would be reported to the Ministry of Agriculture and the animals either slaughtered or tested serologically and carriers slaughtered. In countries other than Denmark, Canada and Switzerland, vaccination of the sows and possibly the finishing pigs would be recommended. The actual choice of the vaccine to be used would depend on those registered for use in the country concerned.

140 (a) You suspect Congenital Tremor Type II. This is caused by a virus of unknown identity. It resembles closely Congenital Tremor Type I or Myoclonia Congenita, the result of intrauterine infection with classical swine fever virus.
(b) For this reason, all cases in which trembling pigs are born should be reported to the Ministry of Agriculture as if they were swine fever.

141 (a) The condition is parakeratosis and is caused by absolute or conditioned zinc deficiency.
(b) Treatment consists of supplementing the ration with zinc, so that 100 ppm is available to the pigs. The lesions will disappear within 10–14 days.

142 Discharges of this type are associated with persistent bacterial infection of the vagina and sometimes of the uterus. The bacteria concerned are often *Actinomyces pyogenes*, a pathogen of the reproductive tract, and others such as streptococci, *Actinobacillus suis*, *Bacteroides sp.* and campylobacters. The infections may be reduced in severity by individual injection with oxytetracycline at parturition or the inclusion of this or similar broad-spectrum antimicrobials in feed or water after farrowing. Treatment of alternate farrowing sows will rapidly allow the effect on weaning to service interval to be calculated.

143 The sow has calcium deficiency. The administration of calcium borogluconate intravenously and the removal of the litter resulted in a complete recovery. This was once a classic time for calcium deficiency to occur, but now it is chiefly seen at farrowing.

144 The animal is a Berkshire. Animals kept in such conditions may be affected by a build-up of worm infections if not treated regularly, and may adopt vices such as chewing stones. They may suffer from erysipelas and avian tuberculosis. Disinfection after any disease is very difficult in such conditions. In populations as small as the Berkshire, inbreeding and infertility play a major part in planning matings.

145 The pig was infected with enzootic pneumonia confirmed by examination of touch preparations for the mycoplasma and by histology. It would have been possible to slaughter the herd and restock from the clean herds used for supply, and to carry out hysterectomy or medicated early weaning. In fact the herd was partially depopulated and treated with tiamulin at 10mg/kg. Disease was eliminated and was not seen again until a fresh breakdown 12 years later.

146 (a) The disease is streptococcal meningitis.
(b) Advise the farmer that the disease could affect man. Outline the early clinical signs to him so that he could treat early cases. Cases of the disease seen alive should be treated with parenteral penicillin and be separated from the rest and given supportive therapy, including water, if unable to drink. It might be worth medicating the ration with phenoxymethyl penicillin, if the number of cases makes it economic.

147 (a) The pig has erysipelas. The skin lesions are pathognomonic and lameness is not uncommon in early infections. The changes in spleen and kidney are not dramatic and might not be noticed in a pig which has died.
(b) The disease may be treated with parenteral penicillin on at least 2 successive days and prevented by vaccination. In breeding stock revaccination should take place every litter.

148 (a) Tail biting may result from overcrowding, poor atmospheric quality or temperature control or from boredom. It is usually associated with one pig, but sometimes more than one is involved. (b) The problem may be overcome by improving the atmosphere, giving animals more space, introducing play chains or straw, correcting the temperature and by using red light or low light intensities so that the blood is not so attractive. The animal(s) responsible can be removed and affected pigs should be treated or slaughtered as appropriate.

149 There are two reasons. The flowering spikes are indigestible and topping encourages the growth of an even and more digestible sward. Topping removes flowering heads in which ergot (*Claviceps purpurea*) might develop within the next few weeks.

150 (a) It is Inclusion Body Rhinitis.
(b) Nothing can be done. It will spread throughout the herd and the gradual development of immunity will protect later generations of piglets. Progressive atrophic rhinitis will not develop.

151 The rhinitis is due to *Bordetella bronchiseptica* infection and pneumonia is a frequent consequence of infection. It is a bronchopneumonia and heals with deep fissuring of the lung. Profuse cultures of the organism can be isolated from turbinates and bronchi. In this case no pasteurellae could be recovered and there was no evidence of IBR. Infection might be treated with oral trimethoprim sulphonamide or ampicillin at 3 days, 10 days and 3 weeks and prevented by vaccination of the sows with one of the atrophic rhinitis vaccines which contains *B. bronchiseptica* antigens.

ANSWERS

Sheep

152 (a) The most likely cause of death is torsion of the mesentery with occlusion of the anterior mesenteric vessels, commonly known as 'redgut' or 'bloody guts'.
(b) Confirmation is by identification of the site of the torsion, which involves all the intestines except for the first part of the duodenum.
(c) It is postulated that the condition arises as a result of the intake of highly fermentable food which passes rapidly along the digestive tract leading to a build-up of gas. Instability of the intestines is followed by torsion of the mesentery. Death follows within a short time (1–3 hours). If seen alive, the animal shows signs of acute colic and severe gaseous abdominal distension. If no torsion is detectable, intestinal contents should be examined for the presence of clostridial toxins.

153 (a) In the UK, the organism most commonly isolated from such cases is *Mycoplasma conjunctivae*. In other countries, *Chlamydia psittaci* has been more commonly implicated and this has been isolated occasionally from cases in the UK. Other bacteria, especially *Neisseria ovis*, may be secondary invaders leading to corneal ulceration.
(b) *M. conjunctivae* is spread from apparently normal carrier sheep, with close contact at feeding, or flies assisting in the spread of infection. Immunity to *M. conjunctivae* is poor.

154 (a) This condition is known as 'woolslip' and is always related to winter shearing.
(b) It is thought to be brought about by high concentrations of cortisol produced as a result of the stress of housing and shearing. High cortisol concentrations have been shown experimentally to cause shedding of the fleece in a similar pattern.

155 (a) Retained placenta occurs only at a low incidence in sheep, in contrast to cattle.
(b) It may be associated with abortion, although many sheep which abort expel the placenta normally. It may also be a sign of a lamb retained in the uterus as a result of dystocia and such animals should be checked for the presence of a retained lamb by balloting the abdomen.

156 (a) This is almost certainly orf.
(b) It may be confirmed by examination with an electron microscope of vesicular fluid or scab material for the characteristic orf virus particles.
(c) Affected ewes may refuse to allow their lambs, which may also be affected by the disease on their lips and gums, to suck. Lambs become stunted or die because of lack of milk, and ewes may develop mastitis.

157 (a) This is strawberry footrot.
(b) Both *Dermatophilus congolensis* and orf virus are commonly implicated, although it is not clear which initiates the condition. It is often associated with grazing stubble or rape and similar crops in wet conditions in autumn.

158 (a) This is footrot which is caused by *Fusobacterium necrophorum* and *Bacteroides riodosus* acting in combination.
(b) Transmission occurs by the introduction of infected sheep or apparently normal carrier sheep into a flock and it spreads rapidly where moist, warm conditions exist.

(c) Control measures include footparing, footbathing with formalin or, preferably, zinc sulphate vaccination and antibiotic treatment. Control should be possible on all farms, although eradication demands determination and hard work.

159 (a) This lamb is suffering from tetanus caused by *Clostridium tetani*. Infection has most likely gained entry at the site of tailing or castration. Treatment is often unrewarding and affected lambs may need to be killed on humanitarian grounds.
(b) Colostral antibodies should protect lambs for 3–4 months, providing that ewes have been fully vaccinated. Unvaccinated ewes should receive two doses of vaccine 4–6 weeks apart, the second dose at 3–4 weeks before lambing is due. Previously vaccinated ewes require a single booster dose 3–4 weeks prelambing. Early and adequate intake of colostrum by the lambs is also vital to ensure good uptake of antibodies.

160 (a) This is gangrenous mastitis.
(b) The common causal organisms are *Staphylococcus aureus* and *Pasteurella haemolytica* either alone or in combination.
(c) An early sign of the presence of the disease is dragging or lameness of the hind limb on the affected side. In some animals the condition is rapidly fatal. Others survive, with sloughing of the affected part of the udder. As this commonly occurs in full lactation, the lambs are likely to suffer severe stunting or starvation.

161 (a) This is a toe granuloma.
(b) It often follows bleeding caused by too severe foot trimming. It may also follow damage by a penetrating foreign body or white line abscessation. If untreated, the hoof will never repair. If simply cut off, profuse haemorrhage occurs followed by regrowth.
(c) These can usually be successfully treated (under local anaesthesia) by careful paring to expose the base of the lesion followed by removal and cautery with a hot iron. Use of a caustic, such as copper sulphate or formalin, may also be successful, but requires repeated treatments.

162 (a) This is a severe orf infection of the tongue and gums.
(b) Unless fed, this lamb will starve to death before recovery takes place. Infection of the teats of the ewe, followed by mastitis is also likely. Human infection may follow handling of these cases unless great care is taken.

163 (a) This is ringworm caused by *Trichophyton verrucosum*.
(b) The sheep were housed in accommodation previously used by calves and infection spread rapidly after the sheep were winter shorn and the flanks became damaged and infected because of the narrow entrances to the building.

164 (a) This is staphylococcal dermatitis (facial eczema) attributed to a coagulase positive, haemolytic *Staphylococcus aureus* which produces an exotoxin.
(b) Infection is spread at feeding, particularly if trough space is limited.

165 (a) This is a case of *Actinobacillus lignieresi* infection. The possibility of caseous lymphadenitis (*C. ovis*) should also be borne in mind, although these cases usually show enlargement of lymph nodes elsewhere in the body.
(b) Actinobacillosis is responsive to antibiotic treatment, whereas caseous lymphadenitis is not.

166 (a) These sheep were affected with maedi-visna (ovine progressive pneumonia).
(b) Diagnosis is by serology [agar gel immunodiffusion (AGID) and enzyme-linked immunosorbent assay (ELISA)]. Post-mortem and histological examination are also helpful. The lungs may be 2–3 times heavier than normal and do not collapse when the thorax is opened. Impressions of the ribs may be visible on the surface of the lungs. Lesions are distributed throughout the lungs.
(c) Affected animals may also show a chronic indurative mastitis. In the visna form of the disease, CNS signs are seen.
(d) Spread of disease is via colostrum and milk from mother to offspring, although horizontal transmission may also occur particularly if sheep are confined indoors.

167 (a) Hill improvement reduces the availability of copper by increasing the availability of molybdenum and sulphur.
(b) On land where lamb growth was normal before pasture improvement, lambs grazed subsequently may show poor liveweight gains, anaemia, weak bones and poor fleece quality. Increased susceptibility to infection may also be noticed. Adult animals on the same pasture are apparently not affected.

168 (a) Although orf virus, mycoplasma sp. and ureaplasms have been associated with some cases, in many, no infectious agent can be identified.
(b) The condition is aggravated by flies such as *Hydrotaea irritans* (headfly) in short docked sheep. In the UK, it is a legal requirement that sufficient tail is left to cover the anus and vulva.

169 (a) This is vaginal prolapse in a heavily pregnant ewe.
(b) Although many suggestions have been made, the aetiology is not clear. Possible factors which may be implicated include large foetal load, body condition (too thin/too fat), bulky forage in the diet, lack of exercise, hypocalcaemia, hormone imbalances. Once the condition has occurred, it is highly likely to be repeated in subsequent pregnancies, therefore culling is usually advocated. A hereditary predisposition has also been suggested.

170 The low birthweight lamb was the result of poor placentation. The most likely sequence of events was the establishment of a mutiple pregnancy (3 or more foetuses), then early death of the other foetuses. If the deaths occur after implantation, the remaining foetuses are unable to utilise the uterine caruncles which would have been occupied by the dead foetuses. Thus, a triplet/quad sized lamb is born. If two embryos from such a litter survive, there may be a marked difference in birthweight of the twins. Overfat ewes also tend to have smaller placentas than ewes which have undergone mild undernutrition in the 2nd and 3rd months of pregnancy.

171 (a) It is essential to ask if bovine colostrum has been fed. The colostrum of certain cows contains antibodies which attack the red cells and their precursors, causing severe anaemia which becomes clinically apparent at 1–3 weeks of age.
(b) Diagnosis can be confirmed by macroscopic examination of the bone marrow, which is creamy white rather than red in colour. There is no other condition which produces this characteristic appearance.

172 (a) This is ventral hernia.
(b) This is often the result of trauma, but may occur as the result of weakness of the abdominal muscles combined with a heavy foetal load.

(c) The animal may become recumbent, in which case it should be killed on humane grounds. If it survives to term, parturition will need to be assisted, since the uterus occupies the hernial sac and there will be insufficient abdominal or uterine contractions to expel the foetuses.

173 Both are manifestations of infection with orf virus. *Figure 199* shows a classic infection around the mouth, which resolves and heals within 2–3 weeks. *Figure 200* shows peristent infection with granuloma formation. Such animals appear to be unable to mount an adequate immune response to the infection.

174 (a) This ram has classic signs of scrapie.
(b) Diagnosis may only be confirmed after post-mortem examination by demonstrating the characteristic vacuolation of neurons in the medulla, pons and midbrain.
(c) Many affected sheep do not show these classic clinical signs and may show a variety of neurological signs, such as inco-ordination, ataxia, excessive nervousness and recumbency, similar to cows affected with Bovine Spongiform Encephalopathy.

175 This is a case of photosensitisation which arises on exposure to sunlight of an animal with photodynamic substances present in the tissues. It arises either by ingestion of plants containing photodynamic substances e.g. *Hypericum*, or because of liver damage which interferes with biliary excretion of phylloerythrin, a breakdown product of chlorophyll. An important cause of this liver damage is the fungal toxin sporidesmin produced by a fungus growing on rye grass pastures.

176 It is likely that one or more of the lambs will fail to obtain sufficient colostrum and so will be vulnerable to hypothermia and infectious diseases. Hypothermia is estimated to be the cause of 30–40% of all deaths in young lambs. The amount of colostrum required for energy provision in young lambs is 210–280ml/kg bodyweight/day, depending on environmental conditions.

177 This is likely to be an infection caused by orf virus. The first sign is usually a blood-filled blister. Medical treatment should be sought, emphasising contact with sheep.

178 (a) This is mycotic dermatitis, caused by *Dermatophilus congolensis*.
(b) Diagnosis may be confirmed by impression smears from the underside of moist scabs, stained with Gram or Giemsa to show the characteristic appearance of the bacterium, which has both coccoid and branching mycelial forms. The same organism may also infect the woolley areas of the body causing classic 'lumpy wool' disease.

179 The common causes of scrotal enlargement are scrotal hernia and orchitis. The swelling should be examined to determine whether only testicular tissue is involved, or whether hernial contents are present. This was a case of unilateral hernia. Both testicles showed hypoplasia as a result of increased scrotal temperature and pressure. Affected rams usually become infertile. The condition is believed to be hereditary, therefore, culling of affected rams and their offspring should be considered.

180 (a) Scouring in very young lambs is caused by a number of infectious agents. Common causes are *Escherichia coli*, lamb dysentery, cryptosporidiosis, salmonellosis and rotavirus. Scouring may also follow incorrect feeding of milk substitutes, although such lambs are often less ill than lambs suffering from an infection.

(b) It is usually not possible to differentiate on clinical grounds, therefore laboratory diagnosis is necessary.

181 (a) This is entropion of the lower eyelid.

(b) If neglected, such cases can develop into severe keratitis with permanent damage to the cornea. Eyes of newborn lambs should be examined for the presence of the condition, which may usually be corrected easily by digital pressure on the eyelid at this stage. If neglected, treatment by injection of antibiotic or liquid paraffin into the eyelid, use of Michel clips, or surgery may be necessary. Since the condition is hereditary, care needs to be taken in selection of breeding stock.

182 A mass of meconium has dried and become adherent to the anal area. This indicates good colostrum intake, but the faecal mass may interfere with subsequent defaecation. It should be removed, taking care not to damage the delicate skin around the anus.

183 (a) This is 'watery mouth' with one lamb in the early stages and the other in a more advanced stage.

(b) Watery mouth does not occur in lambs which have had an early (within 30 minutes of birth) and adequate intake of colostrum. It is associated with the ingestion of *E. coli* and their rapid multiplication in the gut, with the production of endotoxin which damages the intestines causing stasis and build-up of gas. Irreversible collapse probably occurs when the liver is unable to cope with the absorbed endotoxin.

184 (a) This is a case of cerebellar gid.

(b) The signs commonly seen with a cyst in this position are dysmetria, tremor and nystagmus. Absence of the menace reflex, a head tilt and bilateral postural deficits are also associated with cerebellar lesions. Onset of clinical signs and deterioration are often much faster with cerebellar cysts than cerebral cysts because of the much more confined location.

185 (a) This is probably listeriosis.

(b) Diagnosis requires histological examination of the brain to confirm. Serology is not helpful.

(c) Listeriosis has increased in incidence and is particularly associated with silage feeding of sheep. Poorly fermented silage, or that contaminated with soil is particularly dangerous. Infection may also occur in sheep grazing very bare pastures with consequent ingestion of soil.

(d) Infection is thought to gain access via injuries in the mouth or via damaged teeth or tooth sockets, and then travels up the nerves to the brain. It is, therefore, particularly common in young animals which are changing their teeth.

186 (a) This could be Johnes disease. The intestinal wall is thickened and the lacteals are dilated. Some pigmented strains of *Mycobacterium johnei* produce a diagnostic yellow pigmentation of the intestinal mucosa.

(b) Diagnosis may be confirmed by demonstration of *M. johnei* in a smear taken from the intestinal mucosa, or by histological examination of the intestinal wall.

(c) A positive diagnosis may be made in the live animal if the bacteria can be demonstrated in a faecal smear. However, a negative examination does not preclude infection. Serological tests may be helpful on a flock basis. Recent developments in both ELISA tests and with a DNA gene probe are likely to improve the ability to diagnose infected live animals.

187 (a) This is pulmonary adenomatosis (Jaagsiekte).
(b) Affected animals, which are usually 2–4 years of age, show progressive weight loss and respiratory embarrassment. Fluid accumulates in the airways and will flow from the nostrils when the hindend of the animal is raised (wheelbarrow test).
(c) A herpes virus and a retrovirus have been associated with the disease, but only the retrovirus has been shown to produce the disease experimentally.

188 (a) This is probably braxy (*Cl. septicum*), although *P. haemolytica* may also cause acute abomasitis.
(b) Clostridial diseases are largely preventable by vaccination. Colostral passive immunity wanes by 12–16 weeks of age, so lambs retained for fattening or breeding should receive two doses of clostridial vaccine to stimulate active immunity by this stage.

189 (a) This is an interdigital fibroma which arises at the junction of the skin and horn in the interdigital space. There may be unilateral or bilateral growths in one or more feet.
(b) When small, these cause little inconvenience to the animal, but they may become excoriated and infected causing severe lameness. If this appears likely, the growths should be removed under local anaesthesia well before the beginning of the mating season. Since they may have a hereditary component, care should be taken to select breeding animals, particularly rams, which do not show this condition.

190 (a) This is 'daft lamb' disease which appears in some pure breeds as a result of a recessive gene.
(b) The owner should be advised to cull the sire and dam of affected progeny, and other lambs sired by the same ram should not be kept for breeding. Although the clinical signs suggest cerebellar dysfunction, histological abnormalities may not be detectable.

191 The wool fibres show an area of marked thinning about one-third of the distance up the staple from the cut ends. This indicates that the animal received a severe check in wool growth, probably as a result of an acute illness, some weeks previously. This fleece would be downgraded because the fibres would break during any manufacturing process. There is also a narrow band of yellow discoloration between the weak area and tip of the fibres. This may have resulted from a mild attack of mycotic dermatitis.

192 This animal shows abnormally small teat development. This is a feature noticed in infertile ewes which have been members of a large litter, containing at least one male. Crowding of the foetuses in large litters in this breed and in the Cambridge breed appears to lead to placental fusion and production of 'freemartins' as in cattle twins consisting of a male and female. Such animals may be detected by examination of a blood sample for chimaerism i.e. white cells originating in the male sibling.

193 Although several sheep were affected, the absence of pruritis means that causes such as sheep scab or lice were unlikely (although a check should be made for sheep scab if pruritic animals are found). In this case these were healed lesions of an earlier attack of blowfly myiasis (flystrike) which had been treated by the farmer. The maggots cause severe damage to the deeper layers of the dermis destroying the wool follicles. Wool will not regrow on the affected areas.

194 This animal is suffering from 'broken mouth' and premature incisor tooth loss. Periodontal disease with gum recession is present around the remaining teeth, particularly the remaining central incisor. Although there are many theories about the cause of toothloss, such as infectious agents, nutritional and conformation factors and trace element status, no one causal factor has been implicated.

195 This is the result of a non-fatal gangrenous mastitis. Sloughing of the gangrenous area of udder has occurred leaving a granulating area around the stumps of the blood vessels. It is unlikely that healing will occur unless the granulomatous areas are trimmed, but severe haemorrhage is likely unless ligatures are used.

196 (a) This is acute fascioliasis, the haemorrhages being caused by the migrating immature flukes.
(b) Treatment of the whole group with triclabendazole should be carried out and gentle movement to a pasture which does not contain snail habitats. It should be remembered that the lambs will have been infected about 6 weeks ago.

197 (a) There is gross thickening of the intercotyledonary areas and the cotyledons are necrotic, which is typical of enzootic abortion caused by *Chlamydia psittaci*.
(b) The organisms can be demonstrated as masses of red spots in a smear taken from an affected area of the placenta and stained by Ziehl-Neelsen.

198 The most common type of polyarthritis in this age lamb in the UK is tick-borne staphylococcal arthritis or tick pyaemia, but chlamydial polyarthritis is common in the USA.

199 (a) The most likely cause is toxoplasmosis.
(b) It is difficult to confirm the diagnosis, since the typical white spots seen in the cotyledons are not easy to find in cases involving mummified foetuses and, though the ewe will probably have a high antibody titre, this may reflect a previous infection rather than confirming toxoplasmosis as the cause of the abortion.

200 (a) This is chronic fascioliasis, the egg being distinguishable by its large size and golden contents.
(b) Since the whole flock will have been exposed to infection, all the ewes should be treated with a drug which is effective against mature flukes. However, since the flock will have been exposed to infection continuously, it is probably more sensible to use a drug such as triclabendazole, which will also kill immature flukes. A control programme, using strategic dosing in conjunction with the forecast issued by the MAFF, should also be produced. Fluke habitats should be identified and fenced off if practical.

201 (a) These lesions are caused by the headfly, *Hydrotaea irritans*, which are active in mid and late summer.
(b) The most effective treatments are various formulations of synthetic pyrethroids such as deltamethrin and cypermethrin in an oil base, which are applied to the head region but they are not completely effective.

202 (a) The most likely cause is louse infestation, particularly the biting louse, *Damalinia ovis*, but it would be very important to make certain that the sheep were not infected with sheep scab, which is notifiable in the UK and results in much more serious effects.

(b) Although both cause intense irritation and scratching, the lesions caused by lice are not moist but consist of wool loss. Lice may be seen with the help of a magnifying glass and eggs will be found stuck to the wool. Skin scrapings will show the presence of the mites responsible for sheep scab.

(c) Lice are very susceptible to all types of dip; since all the stages of the lifecycle occur on the sheep, a single dipping of all the sheep will control the infestation.

203 (a) The ram has been circling around its box in an anticlockwise direction and the most likely cause is gid, (sturdy or bendro), produced by infection with the larval stage of the dog tapeworm, *Taenia multiceps*, probably in the left cerebral hemisphere.

(b) It would be necessary to carry out a full neurological examination to confirm the site of the cyst before surgery was carried out.

204 (a) If it is assumed that all three ewes are suffering from the same disease, the most likely causes are severe molar tooth disease, Johnes disease or Jaagsiekte.

(b) Examination of the lower jaw externally using the hands and eyes, and the molar teeth with the help of a gag and a torch, should establish whether tooth disease is present. Severe respiratory signs with fluid flowing from the nose if the hindlimbs are lifted will detect Jaagsiekte. Johnes disease is much more difficult to diagnose positively, since the acid-fast bacteria only occur intermittently in the faeces and serology is very unreliable in the live animal. It is probably best to confirm the diagnosis by post-mortem examination (*see* Q186).

205 This is a case of foot abscess, with chronic infection of the outer claw of the hind foot. Infection has obviously been present for some time as rupture of the deep flexor tendon has occurred allowing the toe to tilt upwards. Discharging sinuses are present and there is gross swelling above the coronary band indicating chronic infection of the pedal joint and surrounding tissues. In early cases of pedal-joint infection it may be possible to promote ankylosis of the joint by repeated flushing of the infected area together with antibiotic therapy. Application of a plaster cast will aid healing and prevent such tilting of the toe. In an advanced case such as this, amputation of the digit is probably the best option.

206 (a) Dogs are the definitive hosts for a number of species of tapeworms or cestodes for which the intermediate host is the sheep. The most important are:

(i) *Taenia multiceps*, the cause of gid, in which the larval stage is found in the brain;

(ii) *T. ovis* which has a cysticercus larval stage in the muscles and which results in carcase condemnation in heavy infections;

(iii) *T. hydatigena*, whose larval stage is *Cysticercus tenuicollis* in the liver. The migrating stages of *C. tenuicollis* may cause severe acute liver damage in heavy infections, usually only seen in pet lambs which may live in close proximity to the sheepdog;

(iv) *Echinococcus granulosus*, in which the larval stage, a hydatid cyst, is found in the liver and lungs. Hydatid cysts cause condemnation of liver and lungs and also act as a reservoir of infection for the perpetuation of hydatid disease in human beings.

(b) Dogs should not be fed raw sheep heads or offal and should not be allowed to scavenge dead sheep. They should also be wormed at regular intervals (not less frequently than every 3 months) with a drug effective against cestodes e.g. praziquantel.

207 (a) They are *Ixodes ricinus*, the sheep tick though they are not restricted to sheep.
(b) In heavy infections, they may cause anaemia in young lambs and irritation and damage to the fleece in older sheep and they are responsible for the transmission of tick pyaemia, tick-borne fever and louping ill.
(c) Control is by vaccination (louping ill) and by the application of various tickicidal drugs, by dipping or by pour-on.

208 He has possibly become infected with *Fasciola hepatica* from the wild watercress, which frequently has metacercariae on it from the snails found in the muddy areas in which the cress grows.

209 (a) This is almost certain to be Jaagsiekte or Sheep Pulmonary Adenomatosis, especially as fluid is being produced by the lungs, but it is possible that Maedi or chronic pulmonary abscessation may be responsible.
(b) Post-mortem examination is necessary to establish a definite diagnosis when the extensive tumours with a typical histological appearance will be recognised in the lungs.
(c) No reliable serological test has been produced.
(d) Early recognition of clinical cases and culling is necessary to reduce the extent of the disease in a a flock.

210 (a) Coccidiosis and nematodiriasis should be suspected and a faecal examination carried out.
(b) Although both conditions can occur with little evidence in the faeces at certain stages of the lifecycles, there will usually be at least 100,000 oocysts per gramme of faeces and around 1000 *Nematodirus battus* eggs per gramme.
(c) The whole batch of lambs should be treated with oral sulphonamides, parenteral sulphamethoxypyridazine or oral amprolium/ethopabate for coccidiosis, and with any one of a range of anthelmintics for nematodiriasis.

211 There is obviously serious interference with chewing and swallowing—the most common causes are molar tooth disease and actinobacillosis, which can easily be distinguished by examination of the face and mouth. Unilateral facial paralysis, which occurs in listerosis, may also result in difficulty in chewing and swallowing food, but such cases usually show profound depression and rapid deterioration of their condition.

ANSWERS

Poultry

212   (a) This is intestinal coccidiosis caused by *Eimeria necatrix*.
(b) The condition is usually seen as a flock problem, but occasionally an individual in an otherwise immune flock becomes affected.
(c) It is usually treated with potentiated sulphonamide drugs or a mixture of amprolium and ethopabate in the water.
(d) In broilers, it can be prevented by continuous feeding of an anti-coccidial drug, while in replacement layers, a progressively reducing level of an anti-coccidial drug is included in the feed.
(e) Overcrowding, wet litter and inadequate feed space.

213   (a) This is necrotic enteritis as caused by *Clostridium perfringens* (*C. welchi*) type C.
(b) The causal agent usually inhabits the large intestine and caeca.
(c) Intestinal coccidiosis caused by *Eimeria brunetti* and *Eimeria maxima*.
(d) The condition can be treated by any antibiotic but penicillin in the drinking water is the most effective.
(e) Between 6 and 8% of an affected flock are likely to die if untreated.

214   (a) Ascites/cardiohepatic syndrome/water belly.
(b) Suspected causes include low oxygen tension at the bird level, mycotoxins, toxic fat and lung damage.
(c) The condition usually occurs at 4 weeks but, occasionally, it is seen in individual birds during the first week of life.
(d) There is no treatment that is beneficial at the level of the individual bird. Sometimes changing to mashed feed reduces the incidence but it also reduces the profitability of the flock. Improving ventilation is certainly very useful. One would also check for possible toxins in the feed or litter.

215   (a) This bird is suffering from twisted leg, whose incidence has decreased in recent years.
(b) The cause is not known but it is genetic in origin. The weight of the individual bird has no influence on the condition.
(c) The incidence is reduced by greater physical activity but increased under battery rearing systems. Genetic selection by the primary breeders is the main method of reducing the problem.
(d) Tibial dyschondroplasia, femoral head necrosis, kinky back, rickets, rotated tibias, scoliosis, osteomyelitis, perosis and crooked toes.

216   (a) This is aspergillosis caused by the fungus *Aspergillus fumigatus*. Sometimes *A. glancus* or *A. niger* may be involved.
(b) Lesions caused by this condition may also be found in the air sacs, eyes, brain and spinal cord.
(c) Transmission is by spores from contaminated eggs in the hatchery and from mouldy hay, straw, chaff and feed in the poultry houses.
(d) The very young in all species are susceptible but older ducks are equally susceptible and older turkeys to a lesser extent.
(e) Salmonellosis. Laboratory cultures are essential for confirmation.
(f) Remove any source of the fungal spores, provide good ventilation and cull any affected birds.

217 (a) This is *E. coli* bacteraemia, and polyserositis.

(b) Salmonella septicaemia in young broilers and turkeys, *Pasteurella anatipestifer* septicaemia in ducks and yolk peritonitis in laying birds.

(c) Inadequate ventilation, overcrowding, stress, infectious bronchitis and mycoplasma infections.

(d) The carcase would be totally condemned.

(e) The agent enters via the respiratory system, especially inflamed tracheas.

(f) Any management factors precipitating the condition should first be removed, then use an antibacterial drug initially in the water and possibly follow on with feed medication after determining the sensitivity of the organism.

218 (a) Salmonellosis.

(b) Chronic caecal coccidiosis, chilling and non-specific digestive dysfunction.

(c) Confirmed diagnosis by laboratory culture of the organisms.

(d) Other lesions include blindness, arthritis and pericarditis.

(e) Transmission is via the hatching egg, the hatchery, the environment of the brooding house and feed infected by vermin.

(f) Treatment would normally reduce mortality but would not eliminate the salmonella from the flock as carriers would exist.

219 (a) Aortic rupture.

(b) Erysipelas, pasteurellosis, fowl plague, haemorrhagic enteritis, ionophore poisoning.

(c) There is no successful treatment.

(d) The birds should be kept quiet, sudden disturbances should be avoided and any possibly mouldy hay removed.

(e) On examination, the carcase appears very pale.

220 (a) Duck virus enteritis/duck herpes virus/duck plague.

(b) Diphtheritic oesophagitis and/or cloactitis. Intestinal lesions as annular bands or raised rings. Generalised petechial haemorrhages.

(c) Gross lesions and the clinical picture or virus isolation/duck susceptibility tests.

(d) Although the oesophageal lesions may be regarded as virtually pathognomic of DVE, parasitic infections with the burrowing nemotode *Streptocara crassicauda* or some restricted diets can produce similar lesions.

(e) Usually by migrating feral, ducks coming in onto shared water.

(f) There is no specific treatment but it is possible to vaccinate in the face of an outbreak, if this is done quickly and vaccine is available.

221 (a) This is duck viral hepatitis type 2 (astrovirus).

(b) Commonly young ducklings between 0 and 3 weeks of age are affected, losses between 3 and 5 weeks being complicated by septicaemia. Adults do not appear to be susceptible.

(c) Sudden death of birds in good condition. Opisthotonus.

(d) Serum from recovered birds given intra-muscularly has met with some success. For prevention, day-old foot stab vaccination with live attenuated vaccine.

222 (a) This is duck septicaemia caused by *Pasteurella (Moraxella) anatipestifer*.

(b) Sudden death. Inco-ordination, difficulties in walking and twisted necks.

(c) By culture of the causal organism on blood agar. The organism grows best from brain culture and is slow growing, requiring usually 48-hour incubation.

(d) Clinically, duck virus hepatitis, duck virus enteritis and coccidiosis. At post-mortem, E. coli or other bacterial septicaemia.

(e) Treatment can be difficult in acute outbreaks as mortality may have reached a peak before the appropriate antibiotic can be made available. The choice of antibiotic depends on antimicrobial sensitivity testing with the tetracycline group and sulpha drugs being the drugs of choice via the water.

(f) Predisposing features are any stressful extreme, especially critical stocking density, extremes of cold or heat, a move to different housing or the introduction of sudden shocks such as foxes, etc. Where stress situations may be predicted, the use of preventive treatment with antibiotic in the food may be of benefit.

223 (a) Overscald or barking.

(b) Scald tank temperature too high, line breakdowns resulting in birds remaining static in the scald tank for some time. The problem is made worse by harsh air chilling of dry carcases.

(c) Monitor scald tank temperature. Examine birds at whole body inspection following any breakdown in the scald tank line and trim accordingly.

(d) In cutting plants, remove affected skin. If the muscle is not affected, then the carcase can be salvaged. For whole bird plants only, reject the carcase.

224 (a) Hock burn.

(b) Plantar surfaces of the feet as pododermatitis and breast blisters.

(c) Wet capped litter where ammonia levels can be extremely high just under the surface of the litter. The lesion is caused by direct skin contact. Poor, greasy litter conditions arise as a result of a combination of problems in ventilation, drinker control, poor-quality fats in the diet, etc.

(d) Simple trimming of the shanks can be performed in uncomplicated hock burn. The carcase should be examined for other aspects of poor colour or confirmation.

225 (a) Traumatic damage to the blood vessels of the wing causing subcutaneous haemorrhage. The greening of the lesion is the result of the breakdown of blood pigments. This is not gangrene.

(b) Damage would have occurred on the farm some days before slaughter.

(c) Trim the affected wing.

226 (a) Bile staining from a ruptured gall bladder.

(b) *Salmonella*, *E. coli*, *Campylobacter* or other intestinal bacteria could cause surface contamination of the carcase.

(c) Yes, unless the bile is very freshly spilt and washes off easily under running water. Bacteria will adhere to the skin in a matter of seconds rather than minutes and be resistant to further removal.

(d) Gall-bladder rupture usually results from poorly adjusted automatic evisceration equipment or hand removal by poorly trained personnel. Respectively, adjustment or further training is required.

227 (a) Turkey rhinotracheitis (turkey coryza).

(b) Viral, an avian pneumovirus.

(c) In uncomplicated cases, recovery may be rapid and complete in 10–14 days with low mortality. However, mortality rates can exceed 50% due to secondary bacterial infection, notably due to *E. coli*.

(d) Mortality through secondary infection is made more severe due to physical stress on the respiratory tract associated with other infectious agents (e.g. viruses or mycoplasma), poor ventilation, poor litter control, overstocking and adverse weather conditions.

(e) A variety of avian species show seroconversion, indicating infection. Pheasants may show mild respiratory disease, following experimental infection. Circumstantial and serological evidence suggest swollen head syndrome in broilers and broiler breeders is associated with the TRT pneumovirus.

(f) Single age sites and good hygienic control to maintain stocking density and air quality will reduce the affects of secondary bacterial infection. Strategic antibiotic medication may be useful during stressful periods. A live attenuated vaccine is available for spray administration.

228 (a) Swollen head syndrome (SHS).

(b) Morbidity is usually around 1–2% and rearely exceeds 5%. Egg quality appears unaffected but numbers may fall by up to 10% and hatchability may decrease.

(c) Swelling of the head, notably around and above the eyes. Subcutaneously, there is oedema and purulent underrunning. *E. coli* is easily isolated from these lesions. The ear canal may be blocked with orange discharge. The turbinates are congested. In more chronic cases, egg peritonitis may ensue.

(d) There is circumstantial evidence of seroconversion to the pneumovirus agent of TRT but this has not been proven conclusively. There is no specific treatment but individuals may benefit from removal to a hospital pen, especially if combined with antibiotic medication to control secondary infection.

229 (a) Fowl pox (Avipox) infection.

(b) There are numerous pox viruses within the Avipox genus of the Poxviridae, including pigeon pox, turkey pox, canary pox and pox viruses of birds of prey.

(c) Cutaneous lesions may occur on all areas of the skin where no feathers are present i.e. the head, neck, legs and feet. The so-called diphtheritic form leads to lesions in the mouth, upper digestive and upper respiratory tracts.

(d) Wattle and comb lesions can result from traumatic damage or fowl cholera. Lesions in and around the mouth can be confused with avitaminosis A or trichomoniasis (canker).

(e) Diagnosis is by detection of the virus in scab material, either by direct electron microscopy or the production of characteristic pock lesions on chorioallantoic membranes (CAMs).

(f) There is no specific treatment and if secondary bacterial infection can be minimised, lesions may be self-limiting. Live vaccines are available.

230 (a) Infectious bursal (Gumboro) disease. High mortality has been recorded in commercial laying pullets in rear. Broiler breeder pullets may become sick and scour but mortality tends to be low. Turkeys can be infected but seem unaffected, and other avian species appear refractory.

(b) The bursa is nearly always enlarged in the acute phase of infection and is either deeply congested, as illustrated, or is turgid and oedematous. The plicae may show pinpoint haemorrhages and the lumen of the bursa contain milky or more solid casts. Other typical lesions are ecchymotic haemorrhages in skeletal muscle, notably the thigh and breast, severe kidney damage and pale streaking of the liver.

(c) Agar gel precipitin (AGP) tests can demonstrate the presence of the viral antigen in bursal tissue in the very acute phase and the antibody several days later.

(d) In fully susceptible flocks, infection younger than 14 days can lead to almost total immunosuppression. Gangrenous dermatitis due to clostridial infection may then occur. Later infections cause severe kidney damage and the ensuing litter conditions and may give rise to severe secondary coli septicaemia.

(e) An adequate vaccination programme in breeding pullets should afford 3 to 4 week protection in broiler progeny through maternal antibody. However, highly virulent field strains of the virus appear able to penetrate this maternal antibody and, hence, the strategic use of the so-called 'intermediate' strength live vaccines via the drinking water is recommended in areas of high challenge.

(f) Proventricular haemorrhages are a classical feature of velogenic viscerotropic Newcastle disease virus (VVNDV) infection. The other lesions described at (b) above should help to rule out this notifiable disease.

231 (a) Oregon disease or deep pectoral myopathy.

(b) One or both of the deep pectoral muscles, M. *supracoracoideus*.

(c) Excessive exertion with wing flapping. The sudden exertion results in the need for anaerobic respiration of the muscle to provide a rapid energy source. The resultant acid build up leads to water uptake by the muscle and acute swelling. This swelling in muscle tightly bound by a surrounding fascia causes occlusion of blood vessels and, hence, ischaemic necrosis. The dying muscle initially wet and gelatinous eventually takes on a characteristic green crumbly texture.

(d) Purely aesthetic. This is aseptic necrosis which, unfortunately, is difficult to detect at routine meat inspection.

232 (a) Impaction of the gizzard, also known as MOGPID, referring to the mass of grass protruding into the duodenum.

(b) The condition often arises in newly established free-range systems where birds are given access to lush, long grass and insufficient or unsuitable grit. Pasture management should be such that grass to which hens have access is kept closely cropped. This can be attained by rotating pasture pens with grazing sheep, or by cutting the grass short manually.

233 (a) Infectious sinusitis caused by *Mycoplasma gallisepticum* infection.

(b) Culture of the organism from sinus exudate or serology by rapid slide agglutination (RSA) test, using specific stained antigen.

(c) True vertical transmission via the egg through venereal infection of both the hens' oviduct and stags' semen. Bird-to-bird spread horizontally within a house occurs very quickly via direct contact and is often exacerbated by environmental stress or concurrent bacterial and viral infections.

(d) Eradication is only really achieved by total depopulation of the site. The infection will be well maintained on a multiage site. Control is aimed at the breeding stock level to produce mycoplasma-free eggs and poults. This can be achieved by monitoring breeding flocks serologically. Where positive flocks are detected and cannot be slaughtered, any hatching eggs require treatment by direct egg injection or differential pressure dipping. Progeny can then be used as the nucleus of further breeding stock, being kept in small, separate groups being monitored serologically. Any positive groups should not be used as breeding stock.

234 (a) Nutritional encephalomalacia (crazy chick disease).

(b) Vascular lesions in the cerebellum, giving rise to gross haemorrhages clearly visible in fresh brain tissue.

(c) Newcastle disease virus, Marek's disease, mycotic encephalitis, avian encephalomyelitis and some toxicities.

(d) The condition is prevented by adequate Vitamin E, which may be given in the drinking water as treatment.

235 (a) Avian encephalomyelitis (epidemic tremor).

(b) There are no obvious gross lesions. A viral encephalomyelitis can be demonstrated histologically. Definitive diagnosis involves isolation of the causal picornavirus but this is time consuming and expensive.

(c) Chicks are infected *in ovo* during the acute phase of infection in breeder hens. There may then be lateral spread of the virus excreted in faeces to other susceptible chicks.

(d) The proportion of chicks from immune parents in a mixed source flock placement.

(e) No obvious clinical signs. A fall in egg production of up to 10% may be detected, lasting up to 14 days. Hatchability may fall slightly.

236 (a) Chronic Avian pasteurellosis (fowl cholera) due to *Pasteurella multocida* infection, confirmed by isolation of the organism on blood agar under aerobic conditions. The organism may take 48 hours to grow.

(b) Pulmonary oedema, egg peritonitis or purulent arthritis of the hock.

(c) Carrier birds and rats. The disease appears to be site-associated. There is no evidence of true egg transmission.

(d) Acute infection may be halted by drinking water medication with tetracyclines, but relapses may follow cessation of treatment. Chronic infection may be controlled by in-feed medication with tetracyclines. Killed vaccines are available and may help to reduce incidence on problem sites. Rats and other vermin should be excluded from poultry houses.

237 (a) Lesions caused by rat bites.

(b) Fowl cholera (avian pasteurellosis) problems may follow as acute sporadic mortality or more widespread chronic lameness and external injury.

238 (a) *Salmonella enteritidis* septicaemia.

(b) Although the severe fluid pericarditis lesion illustrated is considered by some to be pathognomic of *S. enteritidis* infection, there is a broad spectrum of septicaemic lesions as polyserositis affecting mainly the heart and liver which may be grossly indistinguishable from other bacterial septicaemias, notably due to *E. coli* infection. Therefore, bacteriological examinations are required for definitive diagnosis.

(c) A variety of clinical manifestations of *S. enteritidis* infection exist. The organism can, in fact, be isolated from birds and their environment where no clinical problems exist. Elsewhere, there are three broad syndromes described. Firstly, high early brooding mortality associated with severe yolk sac infection. Either following on from this or as a separate entity, a clinical picture very similar to that seen with runting-stunting syndrome can be seen at 2 and 3 weeks of age. Stunted birds usually have severe septicaemic lesions. A third syndrome is more insidious mortality, with a high level of condemnations for severe septicaemia at meat inspection.

239 (a) Spondylolisthesis (kinky back).

(b) Vertebral column weakness leading to downward rotation of the sixth thoracic vertebra. The resulting compression of the spinal cord leads to paraplegia and the clinical picture described. The cause is probably multifactorial. There is a definite genotype effect but other factors, possibly rapid early skeletal growth and feed effects have been implicated.

(c) Spinal abscess, osteomyelitis of the caudal thoracic vertebrae or certain myopathies.

240 (a) Syngamiasis (gapeworm) due to the nematode, *Syngamus trachea*.

(b) Fertilised eggs are laid directly into the trachea by adult syngamus worms. These are coughed up and swallowed with the eggs being passed out of the birds' droppings. Following development, larvae or embryonated eggs are either then ingested direct by other pheasants or by earthworms, where the larvae encyst in the transport host, remaining dormant until the earthworm is eaten by another pheasant. Larvae are released and migrate to the trachea.

(c) Mebendazole, fenbendazole or flubendazole can be administered via the feed for 2 weeks, or levamisole via the drinking water for 1 to 3 days. Re-treatment may be necessary as infection spreads slowly through a group. Prophylactic medication is not recommended as birds require the presence of adult worms to stimulate immunity.

241 (a) Chick anaemia agent, provisionally characterised as a circovirus, a member of a novel virus genus.

(b) Disease occurs in the progeny of breeder flocks which only experience challenge with chick anaemia agent during lay. During the viraemic phase, which usually lasts 3 to 6 weeks, the chick anaemia agent is vertically transmitted to the progeny. Limited lateral spread can occur in the hatchery to fully susceptible chicks, i.e. the progeny of other virus and antibody negative breeder flocks. Therefore, breeder flocks infected during rear will be immune prior to lay and will not produce affected chicks. In the case illustrated above, the 2 affected houses were placed with chicks from one young breeder flock, which was also implicated as a source of problem chicks on other recent chick placements elsewhere.

242 (a) Classical Marek's disease, a lymphoproliferative disease caused by a herpes virus. Disease is diagnosed by histological examination of nerves which show typical lymphoid infiltration.

(b) Excess mortality is likely. This may last only a few weeks or continue at a low level throughout lay. Production by the remainder may be satisfactory but less so than that in an uninfected flock.

(c) Apparent vaccination failures may occur related to the vaccination process where errors in the storage and/or dilution of the vaccine or errors in innoculation technique may result in less than optimal dose being given to individual chicks. The presence of residues of other vaccines in vaccine equipment may also inactivate the live Mareks vaccine. There are a variety of host effects including the genetic strain of chicken, maternal antibody interference and interference with vaccinal response by immuno-suppressive viruses. Environmental effects include stress factors such as chilling and overcrowding, field challenge with a virus which may be a variant type not covered by the vaccine or heavy field virus challenge occurring before immunity has fully developed.

243 (a) Erysipelas confirmed by the isolation of the slowly growing Gram-positive *Erysipelothrix insidiosa* from congested tissue.

(b) This is often not established, the disease may be site associated, especially if there is present or previous contact with sheep or pigs. The organism can remain in the environment for considerable time, especially in earth-floor systems and may persist in recovered birds. Vermin may help to contaminate the environment. Outbreaks are often precipitated by stressful conditions including handling, fighting or environmental effects.

(c) Antibiotic medication is only of limited use. The aim should be to reduce challenge and environmental contamination by preventing contact with sheep or pigs and controlling vermin. A combined killed Pasteurella/Erysipelas vaccine is available.

(d) Erysipeloid lesions in man as cellulitis can follow contact with infected turkeys. Infection is usually via cuts and skin abrasions and, in severe cases, can lead to more generalised problems of endocarditis or septicaemia and encephalitis.

244 (a) Histomoniasis, blackhead or infectious enterohepatitis, caused by the protozoan *Histomonas meleagridis*.

(b) The caeca. A necrotic typhilitis is caused by the invasion of the protozoa into the caecal mucosa, which then spreads via the blood-stream, settling in the liver where it sets up further necrotic foci.

(c) *Heterakis gallinarum*, the caecal nematode. *Histomonas meleagridis* is a delicate organism. It is ingested in the caecum by the nematode and infects its eggs. These are shed and will be ingested by earthworms. The organism can then persist in the environment. When these worms are taken in by turkeys, the histomonad is protected in its passage through the bird's intestine until they reach the caecum. Heterakis and the histomonad can infect a variety of avian species including chickens and wild birds, which can act either as reservoir hosts or have previously heavily contaminated ground on which the turkeys are then reared.

(d) In view of the interactions described at (c) above, the use of land previously used for chickens should be avoided. Most commercial turkey rations contain dimetridazole as an anti-blackhead prophylaxis but water treatments can be used in the face of a clinical problem.

245 (a) The nematode worm *Amidostomum anseris*.

(b) The nematode burrows into the lining of the gizzard, notably at the proventricular gizzard junction. Here it causes an erosive haemorrhagic lesion which results in blood loss and inanition. This leads to severe emaciation and anaemia. The lameness reported relates to the marked weakness in severely debilitated birds. Owners are often reluctant to believe this since, unless birds are handled or weighed, they often appear to look in reasonable body condition due to downy feather cover.

(c) Water medication with levamisole or individual treatment of birds with ivermectin by mouth are effective in removing the parasite from infected birds.

246 (a) Haemorrhagic enteritis (HE), an adenovirus infection.

(b) Typical adenoviral intranuclear inclusion bodies.

(c) Agar gel precipitin tests on suspensions of spleen can be used to demonstrate the presence of viral antigen.

(d) Disease is precipitated by a variety of stressors including overcrowding, chilling and nutritional upsets.

(e) Pheasants and chickens. Pheasants dying suddenly in good condition, often show enlarged mottled spleens in which viral antigen and intranuclear inclusion bodies can be demonstrated. Birds appear to die from asphyxia, a consistent post-mortem lesion being severe acute lung oedema. Chickens appear clinically unaffected but infection can give rise to enlarged mottled spleens which may be condemned at meat inspection.

247 (a) Catena lesions, due to so-called catenabacterium.
(b) *Streptococcus faecalis* var. *liquefaciens* infections of the intestinal mucosa allow the catenabacterium to gain access to the blood-stream. The organism settles in the liver giving rise to multiple granulomatous lesions of varying size.
(c) Usually there are no clinical signs. Occasionally in severe infections there may be wasting and debility.

248 (a) Lymphoid leukosis due to avian leukosis virus.
(b) Marek's disease and other leukoses.
(c) Histologically and on the distribution of lesions. For example, Marek's disease commonly causes tumourous infiltrations of the heart and peripheral nerves, tissues which are seldom affected in lymphoid leucosis. In lymphoid leucosis, the lymphoid tumours comprise sheets of immature very uniform cells, whereas in Marek's disease, the cells show marked pleomorphism.
(d) No treatment or vaccines are available. Control is based on using birds from infection-free sources or genetically resistant stock, with hygienic measures aimed at reducing infection from the environment.

249 (a) Infectious laryngotracheitis, caused by a herpes virus.
(b) If infection was introduced to the site by the youngest pullets, then a similar clinical picture would be expected in other susceptible groups on site. For laying birds, egg production may fall dramatically, although quality in the remaining eggs is seldom affected.
(c) The clinical picture described can be virtually diagnostic. The mild form may be less so. Other diagnostic tests include serology (gel precipitin, ELISA, virus neutralisation, pock reduction), virus isolation (pocks on chick embryo chorioallantoic membranes or tissue culture) or histologically by the demonstration of intranuclear inclusion bodies in tracheal exudate or fixed tracheal sections.
(d) Live vaccine may be administered by eyedrop, spray or drinking water. However, a carrier state is induced meaning that on multiage sites, the vaccination programme needs to be continued for all new stock coming onto the premises. The only way to remove infection from a site is complete destocking, with thorough disinfection prior to the introduction of clean birds.

250 (a) Transient paralysis.
(b) Marek's disease herpes virus.
(c) This is an uncommon manifestation of Marek's disease virus infection. There are no significant gross lesions. Histological examination of the brain reveals a typical viral encephalitis, with dense perivascular cuffing with inflammatory cells.

251 (a) Cardiohepatic syndrome, hepatosis or round heart disease.
(b) Unknown. Low oxygen tension, viral and toxic agents have been suggested.
(c) Degenerating hepatocytes, often containing eosinophilic PAS positive cytoplasmic bodies.
(d) Deaths seldom last more than a few days.

252 (a) Infectious stunting syndrome, runting and stunting syndrome, malabsorption syndrome or pale bird syndrome.

(b) Bacteria-free intestinal contents from infected birds will transmit the disease suggesting a viral cause. A variety of virus groups have been implicated including reovirus, parvovirus, enterovirus and togavirus. Poor hygiene, inadequate terminal disinfection and short turnaround times all exacerbate the severity of disease. It is likely that secondary bacterial infection, especially anaerobes, are important in full clinical expression of the disease. In-feed medication of starter rations with antibiotic reduces clinical incidence. Combined infection with *Salmonella enteritidis* or infectious bursal disease causes more severe clinical manifestation.

(c) Loops of small intestine are distended with gas and poorly digested food. Up to 20% of birds show gross evidence of pancreatic atrophy, being most obvious at the closed end of the duodenal loop where the organ may be white, hard and string-like. Histological examination of the affected pancreas shows severe cystic and fibrous change. There is usually a generalised lymphoid atrophy, notably affecting the thymus.

253 (a) Egg peritonitis.

(b) Losses due to this condition are inevitable in any laying flock. However, losses are generally higher in birds coming into production fast. Where the problem persists, this is usually associated with some stress factor. These factors include infectious bronchitis challenge, vent pecking and cannibalism associated with stocking densities and lighting programmes, litter management or general bird behaviour, for example, competition for food as may occur in some floor feeding situations. Treatment requires rectifying the management faults but in-feed antibiotic medication may be required.

(c) Although it is usual to isolate *E. coli* in profusion from liver, oviduct and yolk material, some outbreaks may be associated with *Pasteurella multocida* infection. This would require prompt antibiotic medication to reduce the severity of an outbreak.

254 (a) Avian botulism, due to ingestion of botulinum toxin produced by the bacterium *Clostridium botulinum*.

(b) Feeding on decomposing carcases within the pen or ingestion of maggots containing botulinum toxin. As little as 1 gram of toxin-carrying maggots may be lethal.

(c) Pesticide intoxication through accidental misuse, lead poisoning where there is access to lead shot or yew poisoning, especially through ingestion of leaves during the autumn.

255 (a) Osteomyelitis.

(b) Staphylococci, streptococci, *E. coli*, *Mycobacterium avium* and, occasionally, fungi.

(c) Haematogenous spread from cutaneous infection or more generalised bacteraemia.

(d) Vertebral osteomyelitis commonly affecting the caudal thoracic vertebrae, leading to paraplegia. Infections may arise via haematogenous spread or as a direct extension from an air sacculitis. Mandibular/maxillary osteomyelitis arises from beak injuries or following debeaking.

256 (a) Tibial dyschondroplasia. The condition is perhaps more correctly termed physeal osteochondrosis, indicating a disturbance in endochondral ossification, being replaced by a plug of cartilage of varying size.

(b) The aetiology is uncertain, but is probably multifactorial. There is definitely a genetic component and birds can be selected for low incidence, although in the field situation the incidence from flock to flock varies markedly. Nutritional and environmental factors are clearly important. Rapidly growing male birds appear most susceptible. Continued activity during rapid bone growth is required to stimulate proper ossification.

(c) Mild lesions are usually clinically silent. More severe lesions lead to rotation of the tibia, producing abnormal leg confirmation and obvious lameness, with resulting poor weight gain. In very extensive lesions, the proximal end of the tibia may be so weakened as to lead to severe pathological fracture.

257 (a) Infectious sinusitis associated with mycoplasma infection (*M. gallisepticum*, *M. gallinaeceum*, *M. synoviae* or *M. colomborale*).

(b) Lesions are usually restricted to the upper respiratory tract with the presence of thick, turbid mucus in the infraorbital sinuses and nasal turbinates. In more chronic infections, white caseous plugs may be present in the sinuses with hyperplastic lesions around the external nares. Birds may show loss of body condition or severe dehydration.

(c) Reponse to antibiotics is very variable and often disappointing related to the variety of secondary infections and fact that affected birds are often reluctant to feed or drink. In less severe outbreaks, water medication with tetracyclines or potentiated sulphonamides may be effective in controlling secondary bacterial infections. In more severe outbreaks and in the case of breeding stock, there is little option but to cull any severely affected birds. Treatment of the remainder with a combination of water and food medication with tiamulin appears useful in at least dampening down infection. Veterinarians should be aware that tiamulin can enhance the toxicity of any ionophore coccidiostats being used simultaneously.

258 (a) Scaly leg.

(b) *Cnemidocoptes mutans*, a burrowing mite.

(c) Classical treatment is to soak the feet to soften the hyperkeratinised areas and then apply benzyl benzoate as a parasiticide. More recently oral administration of ivermectin (Ivomec©) has been highly successful in treating individual birds.

259 (a) One-eyed cold.

(b) Probably multifactorial. Infectious components include active mycoplasma or chlamydial infections, simple bacterial conjunctivitis or Vitamin A deficiency. Problems are nearly always precipitated by debility associated with heavy worm infestation or exhaustion after racing.

(c) The success of treatments is usually very variable, probably confirming the variety of causes. The most consistently successful treatment is probably Furazolidone as flock water treatment or for individuals in capsules. Tetracyclines and tylosin treatment can also produce clinical cures. Other managemental and disease problems should be addressed with worming and possible courses of water-soluble vitamins following hard races or late returns from races.

260 (a) Ammonia keratitis.

(b) High ammonia build-up caused by poor ventilation or litter management, exacerbated by any condition causing diarrhoea in the birds.

(c) As well as damaging the cornea, the irritant effect of ammonia may lead to deciliation of the trachea, tracheitis and predisposition to severe respiratory disease by a variety of respiratory pathogens.

261 (a) Synergistic toxicity of tiamulin and ionophore coccidiostat.

(b) There may be little to see other than petechial haemorrhages in fat and pale streaking in skeletal muscles.
(c) Histological examination of skeletal muscle and assay of the ionophore content of the ration.

262 (a) Avian tuberculosis as caused by *Mycobacterium avium*.
(b) Liver, spleen, intestines and bone marrow.
(c) Clinical and gross lesions are strongly suggestive. Crush smears from the chronic granulomas reveal the presence of large numbers of acid-fast bacilli using Zeihl-Neelsen staining techniques.
(d) There is no practical treatment or vaccination. Eradication is not usually feasible due to the weight of the bird and environmental contamination. Control, therefore, can only really be aimed at reducing the effects of infection and removing obviously heavily infected birds. It is possible to detect infection in the live bird. Cultural examination of faeces is hit and miss but injection of avian tuberculin into the wattle can be used to detect infected individuals. These may be culled. When this is combined with a policy of keeping breeding birds for only one laying season, then the effects of the disease can be greatly reduced.

263 (a) Nicarbazin poisoning.
(b) Contaminated broiler or pullet rearing ration.
(c) Fertility and hatchability are likely to be adversely affected.

264 (a), (d) and (e).

265 (a) Adenovirus.
(b) Astrovirus.
(c) Birnavirus.
(d) Paramyxovirus.
(e) Coronavirus.
(f) Orthomyxovirus.
(g) Enterovirus.
(h) Avian pneumovirus.

266 (a) Articular gout, affected joints and tendon sheaths containing pasty deposits of urate crystals.
(b) Renal failure as a result of mineral imbalance, nephrotoxic infectious bronchitis strains or possibly some toxins.
(c) Infectious synovitis due to mycoplasma infection, viral arthritis or staphylococcal infection (bumblefoot).

267 (a) Yolk sac infection.
(b) Starve-outs/non-starters.
(c) Baby chick nephropathy.
(d) Brooder pneumonia associated with aspergillosis.
(e) Carbon monoxide poisoning due to poorly adjusted brooders.

268 (a) Salmonella.
(b) Campylobacter.

(c) Erysipelas.
(d) Ornithosis/psittacosis.
(e) Listeria.

269 (a) i) Collection crates.
   ii)   Water in stunning machine.
   iii) Scald tank.
   iv) Defeathering machine.
   v)   Evisceration equipment.
   vi) All handling by operatives.
   vii) Conveyor belts.
   viii) Badly run reverse flow water immersion chillers.
(b) iii) and iv).

270 (a) Catching.
(b) Crating.
(c) Journey time, ventilation and movement.
(d) Protection from weather whilst waiting at processing plant.
(e) Unloading.
(f) Hanging onto shackles.
(g) Time on shackles before stunning.
(h) Damage to birds on shackles due to collision with stanchion, etc.
(i) Pre-stunning shocks due to water overflow.
(j) Slaughter of unstunned birds.

271 (a) Males and females can be fed different types of feed from different equipment.
(b) To control the weight of cockerels as overconsumption of feed leads to leg problems and reduced fertility.
(c) By placing one of the above over the feed track:
   i)   Toast rack grid.
   ii) Flat wooden board.
   iii) Plastic tubing.

272 (a) House preparation before delivery of the chicks. The house should be clean and well disinfected, adequately littered and pre-heated with ample feeders and water points in place.
(b) Distribution of feed trays and drinkers around the heat source.
(c) Well lit so that birds can find food or water.
(d) Distribution of chicks within a brooder ring related to the heat source. They should be well distributed within the ring. If piled up in the middle, it is too cold, if all to one side there is a draught and if right around the edge and panting, it is too hot.

273 (a) A live microbial feed supplement which beneficially affects the host animal by improving its intestinal microbial balance. Bacterial species commonly used are lactobacilli and streptococci.
(b) A stable gut flora helps the animal to resist infections, especially in the gastro-intestinal tract. They are thought to reduce proliferation and colonisation of pathogenic coliforms in the intestines. Probiotics have been advocated as growth promoters in an effort to replace antibiotics and synthetic chemical feed supplements.

(c) Direct antagonistic effect against pathogenic microbes. Mediated by:
- i) Suppression of bacterial numbers by production of antibacterial compounds, competition for nutrients and adhesion sites.
- ii) Alteration of microbial metabolism by effecting enzyme activity.
- iii) Stimulation of immunity by increasing macrophage activity and antibody production.

274 (a) Obtain raw materials from a reputable source.

(b) Store raw material in hygienic conditions, avoiding infestation by vermin, birds and pests.

(c) Monitor all raw materials for the presence of salmonella before incorporation into final feed.

(d) Feed manufacturing and storage facilities should maintain hygienic practices and avoid infestation by vermin, birds and pests.

(e) All vehicles should be subjected to a regular cleaning and sanitising programme to avoid build-up of waste material.

(f) Finished feed should not be carried in the same vehicles as raw materials.

(g) Vehicles used for loose bulk should either be in closed containers or, if impracticable, should be covered.

(h) Treatment of finished feed with organic acids. This will reduce any residual salmonella contamination and may guard against subsequent contamination of the finished feed.

(i) Pelleting or heat extrusion to reduce residual salmonella contamination. Feed will be susceptible to re-contamination. This process can be used for pelleting and then re-crumbing mash feeds, although the re-mixing machinery should be kept very clean if subsequent re-contamination is to be avoided.

275 (a) i) Botulism due to *Clostridium botulinum*.
- ii) Necrotic enteritis due to *Clostridium welchii (perfringens)*.
- iii) Gangrenous dermatitis and blue wing disease due to *Clostridium welchii* or *Clostridium septicum*.

(b) i) Access to botulinum toxin (usually type C) from decaying poultry carcases, or toxin-carrying maggots. It is possible for there to be toxicoinfection where *Clostridium botulinum* bacteria are ingested and produce toxin in the intestines.
- ii) *Clostridium welchii* in the large intestine is able to proliferate and migrate to the small intestine where toxins produced lead to severe necrotic enteritis. Subclinical *E. acervulina* coccidiosis or digestive problems associated with poor quality grit or sudden dietary change usually precipitate this proliferation.
- iii) Immunosuppressive infection such as infectious bursal disease and chick anaemia agent infection allow cutaneous proliferation of clostridia to produce gangrenous lesions, notably of the wing tips and flanks. Poor hygiene and high stocking rates increase the severity of the condition.

(c) i) Good management and hygiene, especially the frequent removal of carcases.
- ii) In acute outbreaks, water soluble penicillin is very effective in reducing mortality. Anticoccidial prophylaxis, litter control and dietary management all need to be reassessed.
- iii) Adequate protection from early infectious bursal disease challenge in progeny from well vaccinated breeders supplying protective maternally derived antibody. In the case of chick anaemia agent, it is hoped that breeder flocks have become seropositive in rear to protect against viraemia in lay when vertically infected progeny would be produced.

Index

Index

Numbers refer to Question & Answer numbers